WALL PILATES
WORKOUTS FOR WOMEN

28 Day Body Sculpt Challenge Suitable for Beginners & Seniors

Guided Exercises with Videos to Tone Your Glutes, Abs, Back & Lose Weight Naturally

Written by Industry Experts

EVA WELLS & ARTHUR HANSON

© Copyright 2024 - All rights reserved

The content contained within this book may not be reproduced, duplicated, or transmitted without direct written permission from the author or the publisher.

Under no circumstances will any blame or legal responsibility be held against the publisher, or author, for any damages, reparation, monetary loss, injury, or health related issue due to the information contained within this book, either directly or indirectly.

Legal Notice:

This book is copyright protected. It is only for personal use. You cannot amend, distribute, sell, use, quote or paraphrase any part, or the content within this book, without the consent of the author or publisher.

Disclaimer Notice:

Please note the information contained within this document is for educational and entertainment purposes only. All effort has been executed to present accurate, up to date, reliable, complete information. No warranties of any kind are declared or implied. Readers acknowledge that the author is not engaged in the rendering of legal, financial, medical or professional advice. The content within this book has been derived from various sources. Please consult a licensed professional before attempting any techniques outlined in this book.

By reading this document, the reader agrees that under no circumstances is the author responsible for any losses, direct or indirect, that are incurred as a result of the use of the information contained within this document, including, but not limited to, errors, omissions, or inaccuracies.

CONTENTS

	Introduction	1
Chapter 1	Our Shared Goals	5
Chapter 2	Ignite and Unwind	11
Chapter 3	Morning Wall Pilates Routine	25
Chapter 4	Evening Wall Pilates Routine	33
Chapter 5	15-Minute Wall Pilates Routines	40
Chapter 6	Beginner Program: Day 1 – 7	49
Chapter 7	Intermediate Program: Day 8 – 14	57
Chapter 8	Advanced Program: Day 15 – 21	64
Chapter 9	Finish Strong! Day 21 – 28	72
Chapter 10	Hustle and Tone	80
	Conclusion	95
	References	98

INTRODUCTION

SCULPTING THE BEST YOU

Inspiring Those Around Us

"Yeah, I really want to get in shape, but I keep falling off the wagon. It's so frustrating."

I look up from my lunch and see a woman walking along the park's cobblestone pathway. She holds a cell phone in one hand and is frantically soothing down her frazzled hair with the other.

"I just want to look good, you know?" the woman goes on to say. "I'd love a sculpted body, I mean, who wouldn't want to look like a goddess?"

I watch as the woman plops down on the bench next to me. I take another bite of my salad as I listen to her conversation. Today, my Keto-inspired meal is a colorful plate filled with nutrient-rich, low-carb goodness.

"I don't know. Maybe next week I will try hitting up the gym," the woman says, wrapping up her conversation. "Eh, if I feel like it..."

I smile as I chew my lunch, knowing that I have the power to help this woman reach her dreams. I can't help but empathize with her words. Her tone carries a mix of determination and exasperation, a sentiment I've encountered many times.

As soon as the woman ends the phone call, I turn to her and offer a look of kindness.

"I know the feeling," I tell her. "It's not always an easy journey. But you're not alone. We all face challenges on the road to fitness."

The woman glances over, surprised to hear a response.

"Oh, I didn't realize anyone was listening," she says, eyeing me from head to toe. I can see that she is taking in my comfortable yet functional workout attire, my healthy lunch, and the glow I have from my post-Pilates time.

"Do you... Do you have any tips or advice?" she asks.

And, this is what I love to do, I think.

"Absolutely," I tell her. "I have been a personal trainer, a Wall Pilates instructor, and a body transformation specialist for over ten years."

The woman's jaw drops. "Wow. What would you do if you were in my shoes?"

"Consistency is key," I inform her. "Start with small, achievable goals and gradually build up. It's okay to stumble. What matters is getting back up and staying committed."

The woman nods, clearly inspired.

"You know," I go on, "achieving your fitness goals is like taking up a transformative journey. First off, let's talk about the importance of goal setting. Focus on clear goals that resonate with you. They should be your guiding light, motivating you through the ups and downs of your Wall Pilates training."

"That sounds more doable," the woman responds. "I always get overwhelmed when I can't reach a goal."

"Right," I affirm. "It's about making goals that inspire you. Now, as you plot your goals, take a moment for self-reflection. Understand why these goals matter to you. The connection between your personal desires and the power of Wall Pilates is profound. It's not just about exercises; it's about creating a positive change in your life."

The woman cocks her head to one side. "I never thought about the 'why' behind my goals. That makes a lot of sense."

"Now, when it comes to achieving those goals, think actionable steps. Realistic approaches make a big difference. It's not about overhauling your entire life; it's about seamlessly incorporating Wall Pilates into your routine. Sustainability is key."

"That sounds more manageable," the woman says. "I don't want to completely change everything at once."

"Mindset matters too," I say. "Cultivate a positive approach. Your mental focus intertwines with physical progress. Enjoy the journey, relish each movement, and watch how it transforms your workouts."

"I never thought mindset played such a big role. It's usually just about the exercises, isn't it?" the woman responds.

"As you advance, you won't be alone. Progressions are there to challenge you. Imagine evolving beyond the wall, experiencing diverse workouts that keep things exciting. It's about growth, both physically and mentally."

The woman nods. "I like the idea of progressing. Keeps things interesting."

I pat her knee and add, "And always listen to your body. It's your best guide. If something feels off, correct it. Prioritize safety over pushing too hard. Discomfort signals a need for adjustment, not a reason to push boundaries recklessly."

"I've ignored those signals before," the woman shakes her head. "Safety first makes sense."

"Assessing the risk versus reward in each exercise is crucial. Be honest about your limitations. Avoid unnecessary risks, and focus on exercises that align with your capabilities."

The woman stretches out and says, "I've pushed too hard before and regretted it. Being honest about my limits is something I need to work on."

"Training at the right intensity is key," I tell her, "It's not a race; it's a journey. Find a level that suits you. The benefits are immense… more frequent training, quicker recovery, and injury prevention."

"I've never thought about the intensity," the woman wonders, "I always thought more was better."

"Not exactly," I explain. "And, staying consistent can be a challenge. You know, one thing that really helps is keeping your workouts diverse. It makes it easier to stay motivated and actually look forward to exercising."

"Diverse workouts? How does that work?"

I smile. "Well, when your workouts are varied, it prevents boredom," I explain. "You won't feel like you're stuck in a monotonous routine, and that excitement keeps you coming back for more. The more often you train, the better and faster the results."

The woman furrows her eyebrows, taking it all in. "That makes sense. But, isn't it hard to see significant changes in a short time?"

"Not necessarily," I go on. "It's amazing how quickly you can transform your body. I've worked with a variety of people, from soccer moms, to retired senior citizens, to film and television actors, and we've managed to achieve impressive results in less than a month."

Her eyes widen. "Really? How is that possible?"

INTRODUCTION

"No extreme diets or crazy long workouts. It's all about controlled intensity, clean eating, and consistent training. I've seen remarkable transformations in as little as 28 days."

She gasps. "Wow, that's inspiring! How do you keep yourself motivated?"

"Setting clear goals and having a plan helps. Plus, the diversity in workouts makes it exciting for me too. It's like a journey, and every session is a step toward a healthier and stronger you."

"I like the sound of that. Maybe I should give it a try."

And, this is how a person's life can take a turn for the positive, I think.

"Because, it's not just about the destination… It's about the fulfilling journey you create with Wall Pilates. You've got this!"

Finding Your Guide

Just as the woman found motivation and guidance in our conversation, I hope to ignite a similar spark within you, my reader.

Wall Pilates is more than the realm of mere exercises; it evolves into a transformative experience that extends beyond the physical, delving into the core of your well-being.

Think of me as your steadfast companion on new found path, providing more than just workouts…

I am here to be your source of motivation!

Let this journey serve as a radiant beacon of inspiration for you, illuminating the path to holistic well-being. Embrace the challenges that come your way, revel in the victories, and savor every moment of progress.

Together, we will elevate you to new heights in both health and strength.

As we navigate the intricacies of Wall Pilates, you can expect not just physical transformations but an evolution of your entire well-being.

It's more than a workout routine; it's a shared exploration of growth, resilience, and self-discovery.

With each step, celebrate the victories, face the challenges with courage, and relish the continuous progress we achieve together.

This journey is not just about exercises… It's about fostering a harmonious balance between the body, mind, and spirit.

The Origins of Pilates

Before you immerse yourself in the world of Pilates, it is important to know one thing…

Where did Pilates come from, after all?

Created by Joseph Pilates back in the early 20th century and called Contrology at first, this approach focused on connecting the mind and body. Joseph was all about a well-rounded fitness routine, giving importance to strength, flexibility, and endurance.

Now, when we look at how Pilates has changed over the years, it's pretty incredible. In the beginning, as Contrology, it was groundbreaking for emphasizing the mind-body connection. Joseph Pilates envisioned a fitness strategy that not only shaped the body but also built mental toughness.

Fast-forward to today, Pilates has transformed into a widely recognized and easy-to-get-into exercise routine. What makes it work so well is its flexibility, suiting various fitness levels and goals. Pilates gives you a workout that's easy on the body but super effective, involving both your body and mind. The magic lies in the mix of breath, control, and precision, making Pilates suitable for everyone, whether you're just starting or a seasoned pro.

Looking at how Pilates has evolved shows its ability to keep up with the times and adapt to what people need for their fitness journeys.

It's not just a trend; it's a living practice that continues to embrace new ideas while staying true to its roots.

Why Pilates?

Ask yourself: What do you want from this practice?

Is it to shed those extra pounds, tone up, boost confidence, or attain a sculpted physique reminiscent of a goddess?

Acknowledge the genuine desires that fuel your commitment to Wall Pilates.

Consider what may have held you back in the past.

Whether it's time constraints, lack of motivation, or uncertainty about where to begin, Wall Pilates is designed to break down those barriers.

You can expect specially crafted programs in this guide, tailored by an industry expert with over 10 years of coaching and 16,000 hours of one-to-one client experience.

This isn't just a workout regimen; it's a partnership between you and me.

Let's Get Started!

In my role as your Pilates coach, my commitment extends beyond merely leading you through exercises.

Think of me as your workout buddy, offering insights, and keeping things motivating. I'm all about taking our training seriously, but let's make sure to sprinkle in some fun along the way.

Your goals? Well, they're my personal mission too!

Together, we're on a journey to craft the absolute best version of you!

The promises tucked into this book?

They're like magic keys, unlocking your full potential.

Get ready for a ride that's more than just workouts—it's a life-changer.

You're not alone; I'm here to inspire, guide, and celebrate every step of this remarkable adventure with you.

Welcome to the world of Wall Pilates, where each movement is a step towards holistic well-being.

1

OUR SHARED GOALS

"The future belongs to those who believe in the beauty of their dreams."
- ELEANOR ROOSEVELT

Goals are Essential

Many women share the desire to get fit, but a common stumbling block is the absence of concrete goals. Without setting specific objectives, the path to fitness can seem uncertain and overwhelming. It's a prevalent challenge where the eagerness to begin a fitness regimen is often hindered by the lack of a clear roadmap.

Without defined goals, the journey becomes like a ship without a destination, sailing without a specific port in mind. This ambiguity can lead to frustration and, at times, a sense of aimlessness. Many women may find themselves in this position, yearning for fitness but hesitating to establish clear, actionable goals.

Setting fitness goals is like plotting points on a map; it provides direction and purpose to the journey. Without these markers, it's easy to lose motivation and fall short of achieving the desired results. It's not uncommon for the initial enthusiasm to wane when the path ahead seems unclear.

In the realm of Wall Pilates, where sculpting a fit and strong physique is the goal, establishing clear fitness objectives becomes a pivotal step. It transforms the aspiration to get fit into a tangible plan, ensuring that every Wall Pilates session contributes meaningfully to the broader goal.

Think of your fitness dreams as a canvas, and setting goals *without* the rigid SMART criteria as your paintbrush.

It's about understanding why those goals matter, creating a personal connection between what you want and your Pilates practice.

Approach your Wall Pilates sessions with the mindset of someone chasing their dreams. It's not just about going through the motions; it's about actively building the future you envision. Chart your path, figure out what tweaks you need to make to breathe life into your dreams, and let this process shift your mindset. Turn your workouts into a space where the beauty of your aspirations comes alive.

To make the most out of Wall Pilates, embrace the belief in your dreams, just like Eleanor Roosevelt suggests. This mindset injects purpose into every stretch, pose, and routine, making each session a journey toward the beauty you dream of. In Wall Pilates, your goals are crafted by your dreams, and your results are created by your consistent actions over time.

Aspire, Achieve, Advance: Goals Get Harder with Time

As we kick off this journey, consider what shifts you can make… what aspects of your routine can change, and what improvements you aim to achieve. These goals will be the milestones that shape our path, providing direction to your Wall Pilates practice.

Approaching your Wall Pilates training with the right mindset is key. It's not just about physical exertion; it's about a mental shift. Cultivate a mindset of determination, resilience, and a commitment to growth.

Each session becomes an opportunity to not only challenge your body but also elevate your mental fortitude.

But here's the beauty of our journey... it evolves!

As you progress, as you become more adept in your Wall Pilates practice, we won't just maintain the status quo. Instead, I'll introduce progressions that keep pushing your boundaries. Advanced program progressions will be like unlocking new levels in a game, challenging yet exhilarating.

In each 28-day training cycle, the goal is not just repetition but progression. You'll experience tailored challenges that match your evolving skill level. Some of the advanced program progressions might even take you away from the wall, offering a chance to explore new dimensions in your Pilates practice.

This dynamic approach ensures that every cycle is a step forward, a step closer to your fitness aspirations. It's not just about the physical exertion; it's about the joy of discovery, the thrill of pushing limits, and the satisfaction of achieving more than you thought possible.

So, let's set those Pilates goals, embrace the challenges, and together, sculpt a journey that goes beyond the expected, into the extraordinary world of Wall Pilates.

Example Goals that Get Harder with Time

Beginner Stage (Days 1-7):
- Goal: Complete a 15-minute Wall Pilates routine incorporating foundational exercises.
- Daily Goal: Increase daily step count by 2,000 per day and track it through your smart device. Add 1 set of 25 squats before breakfast.
- Focus: Establish a consistent workout routine, emphasizing proper form and building endurance.

Intermediate Stage (Days 8-14):
- Goal: Enhance the 15-minute routine with intermediate-level exercises.
- Daily Goal: Continue with the increased daily step count and morning squats. Add a 30-60 second plank and 1 set of 15 tricep dips before dinner.
- Focus: Increase complexity, refine technique, and introduce variations to challenge the body.

Advanced Stage (Days 15-21):
- Goal: Execute an advanced 15-minute Wall Pilates routine, incorporating dynamic and challenging movements.
- Daily Goal: Maintain the daily step count, morning squats, plank, and tricep dips. Add drinking over 2 liters of water per day.
- Focus: Improve fluidity, precision, and intensity in each exercise, pushing beyond previous boundaries.

Finish Strong! (Days 21-28):
- Goal: Master a 15-minute routine that seamlessly combines advanced exercises for a comprehensive workout.
- Daily Goal: Sustain the daily step count, morning squats, plank, tricep dips, and adequate water intake.
- Focus: Fine-tune every movement, emphasizing control, balance, and a deeper mind-body connection.

A Symphony of Safety: No Exercise Worth the Risk

I often think back to the first time one of my Wall Pilates participants forgot to listen to her body.

It was a normal weekend morning, and I was guiding the class through a series of invigorating exercises. The soothing melody providing a backdrop to the graceful movements against the wall.

Among the participants, Sarah caught my attention as she pushed herself fervently, seemingly oblivious to the subtle signals her body was sending.

I knew I had to do something.

So, approaching Sarah with genuine concern etched on my face, I urged her to ease up on the intensity.

"Listen to your body," I advised gently, emphasizing the importance of adjusting the posture and moving at a pace that felt right for her.

The class paused, awaiting Sarah's response.

"I am!" she insisted. "I am!"

Despite my guidance, Sarah, determined to keep up with the group, persisted with the demanding routine. It was a pivotal moment when, attempting a challenging pose, she winced in pain, a clear indication that she had pushed herself beyond her limits.

Swiftly guiding her to a gentler position, I reinforced the lesson: "This is why it's crucial to listen to your body. Adjust, take it slow, and ensure each movement feels right for you."

As the class resumed, I continued to stress the significance of tuning into one's body, turning a moment of discomfort into a valuable lesson that would resonate long after the session concluded.

When you start Wall Pilates, think of it as having a conversation with your own body. You need to tune in to the unique language it speaks, feel the rhythm, and respond to the subtle cues it shares. Just like a heart-to-heart chat, listening to your body is important when it comes to Pilates.

Think of it as getting to know a good friend. Your body has a lot to say, and it's not just noise... It's a guide, a companion in this fitness exploration. So, we're talking about more than just hearing what your body has to say; it's about truly understanding and respecting its voice.

As you flow through each Pilates move, pay attention to those little signals, those twinges, those moments of ease. They're not random; they're your body communicating, giving you a heads up. It's like your body saying, "Hey, let's do this together, but here's what I need."

Listening to your body doesn't mean that your workouts should feel easy. Your workouts should push you to a level that feels tough but controlled. This will make your muscles adapt to the training overload you're placing on it by developing a sculpted and lean body.

This isn't a solo performance; it's a duet between your intentions and your body's responses. You should make Pilates practice a dialogue, a conversation where every move is a word, and every routine is a story. Because in Wall Pilates, listening isn't just a skill; it's the secret sauce to unlocking the full potential of your journey to wellness and achieving the outstanding physical results or physique you desire.

How to Listen to Your Body: Step-by-Step

1. Mindful Awareness: Begin by cultivating mindful awareness during your Wall Pilates practice. Tune into your body's sensations, acknowledging any tightness, discomfort, or ease.
2. Breath Connection: Pay attention to your breath. It should be steady and in sync with your movements. If you find yourself holding your breath or experiencing shortness of breath, it's an indicator to modify your intensity.

3. Check-In Periodically: Take brief pauses between exercises to check in with your body. Notice how different muscle groups feel, and be attuned to any areas of tension or strain.
4. Scale of Comfort: Implement a scale of comfort. On a scale of 1 to 10, assess the level of comfort with each movement. Aim for a range between 5 and 7, avoiding extremes. If you find yourself consistently above this range, consider adjusting the exercise.
5. Modify Intensity: Don't hesitate to modify the intensity of each movement. Whether it's reducing the range of motion or using a support prop, adapting the exercises to suit your current fitness level is crucial.
6. Pain vs. Discomfort: Distinguish between pain and discomfort. Discomfort is a natural aspect of challenging your body, but pain is a signal to stop. If you experience sharp or persistent pain, cease the exercise immediately.
7. Honest Self-Assessment: Engage in an honest self-assessment of your physical condition. If you're fatigued, consider whether pushing through is beneficial or if a gentler approach would be more appropriate.
8. Fluid Transitions: Ensure your movements have a fluid quality. Jerky or forced motions may indicate that you're exceeding your body's current capacity. Aim for smooth transitions between exercises.
9. Post-Workout Reflection: After completing your Wall Pilates routine, take a moment for post-workout reflection. Note how your body feels overall and if there are specific areas that require attention or modification in future sessions.
10. Consistent Communication: Establish a consistent line of communication with your body. It's an ongoing dialogue that evolves with each session. By actively listening and responding, you empower yourself to derive maximum benefit from your Wall Pilates practice while minimizing the risk of injury.

Creating Your Ideal Wall Pilates Space

Starting a Wall Pilates exercise plan is not just about the exercises; it's about setting the stage for a dedicated and harmonious practice. Creating an ideal space for Wall Pilates can significantly enhance your experience, allowing you to focus, move freely, and immerse yourself in the mind-body connection.

Here's a guide to help you craft the perfect environment for your Wall Pilates sessions:

Choose an Open Wall Space

Select a wall with ample space where you can move freely without any obstructions. Ensure the area is clear of furniture or potential hazards, providing a safe and uncluttered canvas for your exercises.

Gather Essential Equipment

While Wall Pilates doesn't require extensive equipment, having a few essentials can enhance your practice. Invest in a quality yoga mat for comfort and stability. If you're incorporating props, such as resistance bands or light weights, keep them within reach for easy access during your sessions.

Enhance Lighting and Ambiance

Optimize natural light whenever possible, as it can contribute to a positive and energizing atmosphere. If practicing in the evening, consider adding soft, ambient lighting to create a calming environment. A well-lit space not only improves visibility but also sets the mood for focused and mindful movement.

Designate a Dedicated Pilates Corner

Create a designated corner or section of the room specifically for your Wall Pilates practice. This signals to your mind that it's time to transition into your workout routine, fostering a sense of commitment and routine.

Personalize Your Space

Infuse your Wall Pilates area with personal touches that inspire and motivate you. Whether it's uplifting quotes, vibrant colors, or elements of nature, incorporating elements that resonate with you can enhance your connection to the practice.

Ensure Proper Ventilation

Good air circulation is essential for a comfortable and invigorating workout. Ensure your chosen space is well-ventilated, allowing fresh air to flow during your sessions. Consider opening windows or using a fan to maintain a pleasant environment.

Minimize Distractions

Create a focused and distraction-free zone by minimizing external disruptions. Silence your phone, choose a time when household activity is minimal, and communicate your intention to practice undisturbed during specific periods.

Establish a Routine

Consistency is key in any fitness journey. Set a regular schedule for your Wall Pilates sessions, helping you establish a routine that aligns with your daily rhythm. Having a predictable practice time enhances commitment and facilitates long-term adherence to your goals.

Elements of an Ideal Wall Pilates Room:

Quality	Good Example	Poor Example
Ample Wall Space	Features a clear and open wall space free from obstructions.	Limited or cluttered wall space hinders movement and exercise execution.
Quality Flooring	Equipped with a comfortable and supportive floor surface, such as a yoga mat or padded flooring.	Hard or uncomfortable flooring that may impede the comfort and safety of exercises.
Essential Equipment	Provides easy access to necessary Pilates props like resistance bands or light weights.	Lacks essential equipment, making it challenging to perform a variety of exercises.
Optimal Lighting	Well-lit with natural or ambient lighting to create a positive and energizing atmosphere.	Poor lighting hinders visibility and the overall experience.
Personalization	Personalized with motivational elements, such as quotes, colors, or decor that resonate with the individual.	Lacks personal touches, potentially diminishing motivation and connection to the practice.

Proper Ventilation	Well-ventilated with good air circulation for a comfortable and refreshing workout.	Poor ventilation leads to discomfort during exercises.
Distraction Free Environment	Minimizes external disruptions, providing a focused and distraction-free zone.	High potential for disturbances, such as noise or interruptions, affecting concentration.

By thoughtfully curating your Wall Pilates space, you're not just creating a physical area; you're cultivating a sanctuary for self-improvement and holistic well-being. This intentional approach to your practice environment ensures that you will enter each session with a mindset purely focused on the exercises ahead, and the results you want.

Concluding Thoughts:
Unveiling the Power of Preparation in Your Wall Pilates Journey

Optimizing your Wall Pilates experience involves not only setting concrete goals but also recognizing the critical importance of mental and physical preparation before each workout. As we transition into this pivotal phase, let's look deeper into the essence of connecting with your breath. The upcoming sections promise to unravel the intricacies of this fundamental element, providing you with a comprehensive yet succinct understanding of its profound impact.

Within these pages, you will find illuminating examples of warm-up routines, shedding light on why allocating time to this practice is paramount for elevating your workout sessions and expediting visible results. The exploration extends to the profound connection between warm-ups, the engagement of your mind with your muscles, and the subsequent metabolic implications. Our journey will further venture into the realm of dynamic stretches, accentuating their role in priming your body for optimal performance.

As this chapter culminates, the focus gracefully shifts to the crucial aspects of cooling down and incorporating static stretches. Here, we will unravel the role these practices play in hastening recovery, nurturing muscle development, and sculpting a physique that embodies both leanness and flexibility. Anticipate an insightful exploration into unlocking the full spectrum of benefits that your Wall Pilates routines have to offer. Stay tuned for a journey that promises to enhance your understanding and maximize the rewards of your Pilates practice.

2

IGNITE AND UNWIND
THE ESSENTIAL WARM-UP AND COOL-DOWN RITUALS

"Flexibility is crucial to my fitness. Incorporating a good warm-up and cool-down into every session decreases my chances of injury."

— SAMANTHA STOSUR

"Great effort, everyone! Let's focus on engaging those core muscles as we move through the exercises," I cheer on the group of people as they begin the routine.

Bright sunlight streams through the studio's large windows, making it a perfect day for Wall Pilates. The room is alive with energy, mats neatly aligned against the wall, and eager faces ready for the session.

As we progress, I notice that one of my regular participants seems to be struggling to grasp the moves.

That's strange, I think, *Lucy is always on top of her game!*

So, I approached her with a supportive smile, "Hey, Lucy, is everything okay? I noticed you seem a bit unsure about the moves," I inquire, my concern evident in my tone.

She hesitates before admitting, "Honestly, Eva, I'm just not feeling into it today."

Understanding that motivation can fluctuate, I crouch down to her eye level, maintaining an empathetic gaze.

"That's completely okay, Lucy. We all have those days. Let's take a moment to explore why you might be feeling this way," I suggest, creating a safe space for her to share.

After a thoughtful pause, Lucy opens up, "I guess I'm just not mentally here. My mind is all over the place today."

Nodding understandingly, I proceed to explain, "You need to prepare your mind and body before you workout. In order to do that, we need to have three things."

Lucy's eyes widen. "What are they?"

I grin. Holding up my hand, I count off each item with my fingers.

"First, you need to connect your mind and breath with your body. Second, you need an excellent warmup. And, you need to prepare for a great cool-down session."

Lucy tilts her head to one side. "What do you mean by connecting my mind and breath with my body?"

"Our mental state plays a crucial role in our workout experience. That's why I emphasize the importance of preparing your mind and body before each session. Let's focus on connecting with your breath."

She nods and squares her shoulders, ready to follow my lead.

"Close your eyes and take a deep breath in, feeling the air fill your lungs. As you exhale, imagine releasing any tension or distractions. This simple act helps center your thoughts and brings a sense of calm."

I continue, "Connecting with your breath is not just about the physical aspect; it's a gateway to mindfulness. By syncing your breath with movement, you create a powerful mind/body connection. It enhances concentration, reduces stress, and makes your workout more effective."

Encouraging her to give it a try, I add, "Feel the rhythm of your breath guide your movements. It's like a dance between your mind and body. When you're mentally present, the physical benefits follow suit. Let's take it one step at a time, while keeping in mind that Wall Pilates is as much about the mind as it is about the body."

With a supportive smile, I guide Lucy back into the flow of the class, ensuring she feels empowered to reconnect and find her rhythm.

Lucy takes a moment to absorb the guidance, and as the class continues, I periodically check in on her, offering additional encouragement. After a few minutes, I approach her again, making sure she feels comfortable and supported.

"Feeling a bit more centered now, Lucy?" I ask, my tone conveying both reassurance and motivation.

She nods, offering a small smile. "Yeah, thanks, Eva. That breathing exercise really helped."

I acknowledge her progress with a warm smile, "You're doing great. Try to focus on more than just the physical workout; it's about the mind-muscle connection too. When you engage your mind in each movement, it intensifies the benefits. It's like sculpting your body from the inside out."

As we head deeper into the session, I elaborate on the concept of mind-muscle connection. "Think of it as a conversation between your mind and the specific muscle you're working. Visualize the muscle contracting and releasing with each movement. This not only enhances the effectiveness of the exercise but also creates a more mindful and intentional workout experience."

Transitioning seamlessly, I guide Lucy into understanding the importance of a great warm-up.

"Now, let's talk about the warm-up. It's not just about preparing your body physically; it sets the tone for the entire session. Dynamic stretches increase blood flow, improve flexibility, and activate the muscles we'll be focusing on during the workout. It's like priming your body for the main performance."

We proceed to discuss the significance of a great cool-down. "And, of course, a great cool-down is equally important. It helps your body recover faster, reduces muscle soreness, and promotes flexibility. It's like giving your muscles a well-deserved moment to relax after the intense work they've done."

Encouraging Lucy to incorporate these elements into her routine, I emphasize, "So, whether it's the mind-muscle connection, a dynamic warm-up, or a soothing cool-down, each component contributes to a holistic and fulfilling Wall Pilates experience. It's about taking care of your body and mind, allowing them to work in harmony for your overall well-being."

The class continues with renewed energy, and Lucy, now more connected and engaged, begins to find her rhythm within the mindful movements of Wall Pilates.

Lucy's experience is something many of us encounter at different points in our fitness journeys. It's crucial for anyone stepping into the realm of Wall Pilates to recognize that preparing the mind and body is an essential foundation for a fulfilling workout. Whether you're a seasoned practitioner or a beginner, taking a moment to connect with your breath gets you ready for a mindful and focused experience. Incorporating a thorough warm-up primes your body for the challenges ahead, enhancing flexibility and blood flow. Equally important is the cool-down, offering a gentle conclusion that aids in recovery and flexibility.

These three elements, *connecting your breath, warming up, and cooling down*, are not just rituals; they are the pillars that ensure a holistic and effective Wall Pilates practice.

So, as you continue, consider how you'll integrate these elements into your routine, creating a harmonious balance between mind and body in every session.

Breath as Your Guide: Navigating Pilates with Mindful Precision

Connecting with your breath is a fundamental aspect of unlocking the full potential of your Pilates practice. The key to achieving a sense of harmony and bliss during your Pilates routine lies in understanding the intimate connection between breath and movement. In an article featured on *Pilates Reformers Plus,* it is explained that "the rhythm and depth of your breath can greatly influence the effectiveness of each exercise, making it an essential aspect of your overall experience."

In Pilates, proper breathing techniques are not merely a formality but a crucial tool for creating a strong mind-body connection. By directing your attention inward and focusing on the inhale and exhale, you become more attuned to the sensations in your body. *Pilates Reformers Plus* notes, "This heightened awareness allows you to make subtle adjustments and maintain control throughout the exercises." The act of connecting with your breath serves as a guide, helping you navigate through each movement with precision and mindfulness.

Moreover, synchronized breathing promotes efficient oxygen flow to the muscles, nourishing and energizing them for optimal performance. The article explains, "Deep inhalations bring fresh oxygen into the bloodstream while exhaling eliminates waste products like carbon dioxide." This exchange not only enhances physical capabilities but also prevents unnecessary tension or strain that may arise from holding one's breath during challenging movements. The conscious connection with breath becomes a vital component in creating a Pilates experience that is both effective and sustainable.

Incorporating breath awareness into your Pilates routine goes beyond the physical benefits; it extends into the realm of stress management and relaxation. By taking deep breaths and focusing on the present moment, you cultivate a calm state of mind. *Pilates Reformers Plus* suggests, "Using breath to manage stress and promote relaxation is an essential aspect of integrating mindful practices into daily life." This intentional breathing technique triggers the parasympathetic nervous system, facilitating rest and relaxation. Therefore, connecting with your breath in Pilates becomes a holistic approach, enriching not only your physical performance but also fostering your mental well-being.

How to Connect your Breath with your Body

- Mindful Beginnings: Start your Pilates session with a moment of conscious awareness. Close your eyes, focus on your breath, and be present in the moment.
- Diaphragmatic Breathing: Practice deep diaphragmatic breathing by inhaling through your nose, expanding your lower abdomen, and exhaling slowly through pursed lips, engaging your core.
- Movement Synchronicity: Coordinate your breath with movements. Inhale during preparation, exhale during exertion. This synchronization enhances control and flow.
- Rib Expansion: Expand your ribcage outward during inhalation. Feel the expansion without lifting your shoulders and exhale slowly while maintaining this position.
- Segmented Breathing: Divide your torso into sections: upper chest, middle ribs, and lower belly. Inhale sequentially from bottom to top, exhale in reverse order.
- Mindful Transitions: Stay attuned to your breath during transitions between exercises. Inhale deeply as you prepare, exhale fully as you initiate the next movement.
- Paced Breathing: Experiment with rhythmic breathing, inhaling for a count and exhaling for a longer count. This promotes calmness and distraction from discomfort.

- o Breath Holds: Integrate short breath holds at movement peaks for added challenge, focus, and deeper engagement of core muscles.
- o Progressive Integration: Gradually include breath awareness throughout your routine. Dedicate a few minutes at the session's start or end to focused breathing.
- o Listen to Your Body: Adjust your breathing to match exercise intensity. Ensure it complements your movements, fostering a harmonious connection between breath and body.

Unlocking the Power of Pilates Warm-Up: A Comprehensive Guide

Getting the maximum results out of your Wall Pilates program necessitates more than just enthusiasm; it requires a strategic approach to preparation. In her article, "10 Essential Pilates Warm-Up Exercises", April Benshosan emphasizes, "A proper warmup before exercise makes your muscles and joints more mobile, gets your circulation going, and improves your body's neuromuscular communication and control." The significance of a well-structured warm-up routine before delving into Pilates lies in its ability to optimize performance, accelerate results, and foster a profound mind-muscle connection.

Warming up is not an arbitrary ritual but a prerequisite for unlocking the full potential of a Pilates session. In the words of *Phitosophy*, "Going into Pilates entirely unprepared would be counterintuitive." It primes the body for the challenges ahead, gradually awakening each muscle group. In the absence of a proper warm-up, the body may struggle to reach its peak performance state, hindering the effectiveness of the Pilates experience.

The duration of a Pilates warm-up is not measured in rigid minutes but in the intentional engagement of key exercises. As Phitosophy suggests, "Just try a few simple exercises the morning or evening before your class, and note the improvements in your workout performance." Pilates warm-ups often involve a series of dynamic stretches and movements that span a brief yet impactful timeframe. Allocating 10-15 minutes to these purposeful exercises ensures a comprehensive warm-up without unnecessary prolongation.

The benefits of a warm-up extend beyond mere preparation; they significantly enhance the overall Pilates workout. Engaging in targeted stretches, such as Pilates imprinting, arm reach-and-pull, and pelvic thrust exercises, contributes to increased mobility, improved neuromuscular communication, and enhanced circulation. April Benshosan, in her article on essential Pilates warm-up exercises, highlights how these exercises open up hip flexors and chests, which is crucial for the demands Pilates places on the core.

How do we Engage our Core?

Engaging the core involves contracting and activating the muscles in the abdominal region. To do this, envision pulling your belly button towards your spine while maintaining normal breathing. This action stabilizes the spine, promoting better posture and reducing the risk of lower back pain. When engaging the core, you should feel a subtle tightening in the abdominal muscles, indicating their activation. This practice is crucial for overall strength and stability, supporting daily movements and preventing injury. By consistently incorporating core engagement into exercises and daily activities, you build a strong foundation for improved balance, posture, and a resilient spine.

How do we Ensure a Neutral Spine?

Engaging a neutral spine in wall Pilates involves aligning your spine with the wall, maintaining its natural curves. To achieve this, focus on keeping the back of your head, shoulders, and hips in contact with the wall. This promotes proper spinal alignment and reduces strain on the neck and lower back. Engaging a neutral spine is essential for distributing forces evenly throughout the body during Pilates exercises, optimizing muscle engagement and minimizing the risk of injury. When doing so, you should feel a gentle connection between your spine and the wall, ensuring a stable and supported posture that enhances the effectiveness of the workout and contributes to long-term spinal health.

Consistent Pilates practice coupled with a well-executed warm-up expedites the journey toward desired results. April Benshosan emphasizes the importance of intentional breaths, stating, "In Pilates, you use intentional breaths to get more out of each exercise. It helps keep you relaxed and deliver oxygen most efficiently to your working muscles." The improved muscle activation, flexibility, and control achieved through a thoughtful warm-up translate into accelerated progress and more pronounced results over time.

At the core of Pilates is the concept of the mind-muscle connection, a symbiotic relationship between mental focus and physical movement. A thorough warm-up, such as the Pilates imprinting and arm reach-and-pull exercises, serves as a bridge to establish and fortify this connection. It allows individuals to tune into their bodies, promoting awareness, control, and precision in each movement.

When practicing Wall Pilates, a warm-up is not a mere formality but a necessity that prepares your body and unlocks its ability to move through full range, while engaging the muscles you're targeting. Embrace the warm-up as a key part of your Wall Pilates workout session, and trust that it will help to accelerate your results, and to strengthen your mind-muscle connection.

Example Wall Pilates Warm-Up Exercises: Harnessing the Power Within

These Wall Pilates warm-up exercises combine the support of the wall with dynamic stretches, providing a foundation for a mindful and effective Wall Pilates session. Incorporate these movements into your routine to optimize your warm-up and establish a strong mind-muscle connection.

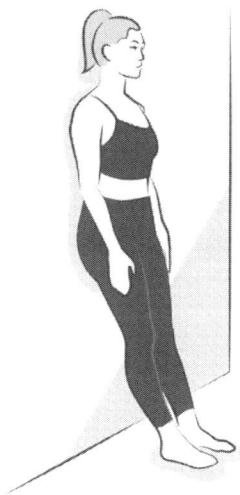

Pilates Imprinting against the Wall

Stand with your back against the wall, ensuring a neutral spine. Gently engage your core, allowing your spine to imprint against the wall.

Inhale deeply through your nose and exhale slowly through your mouth.

Feel the lengthening of your spine against the wall, promoting mindfulness and alignment.

Sets and Repetitions: Perform 2 sets of 10 repetitions.

Targets: Core muscles and spinal alignment.

Purpose: This exercise focuses on creating a neutral spine against the wall, engaging the core for stability.

What to Feel: As you engage your core and allow your spine to imprint against the wall, focus on feeling the gentle lengthening of your spine. Connect with the wall to promote mindfulness and precise spinal alignment throughout the movement.

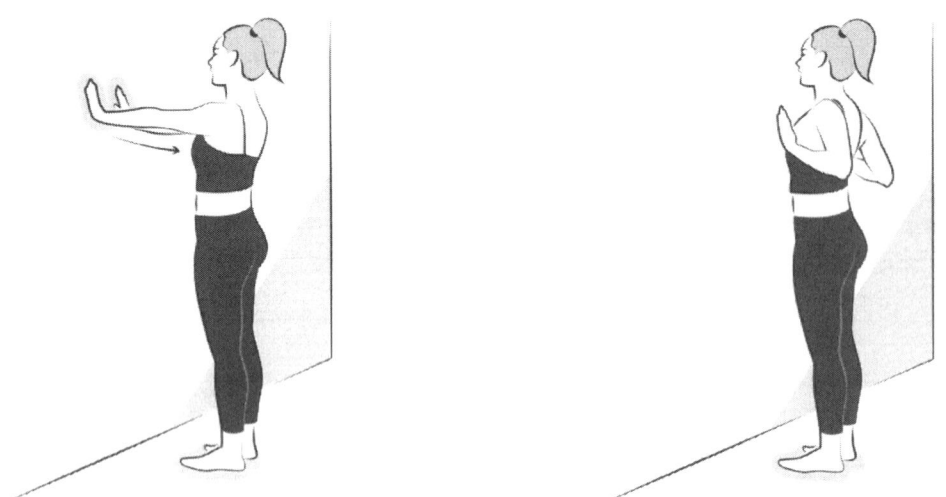

Arm Reach-and-Pull with Wall Support

Stand with your feet shoulder-width apart, facing the wall. Lift your arms straight in front of you, keeping your wrists up and fingers loose. Inhale as you reach forward, opening your shoulder blades. Exhale as you pull your arms back, engaging your shoulders and maintaining arm extension.

Sets and Repetitions: Complete 3 sets of 12 repetitions.

Targets: Shoulders, arms, and upper back.

Purpose: This exercise aims to improve shoulder and arm strength while maintaining proper form against the wall.

What to Feel: During the reach, focus on opening your shoulder blades against the wall, feeling a gentle stretch. As you pull your arms back, concentrate on engaging your shoulders and maintaining full arm extension. Pay attention to the controlled movement and the sensation in your shoulder and upper back muscles.

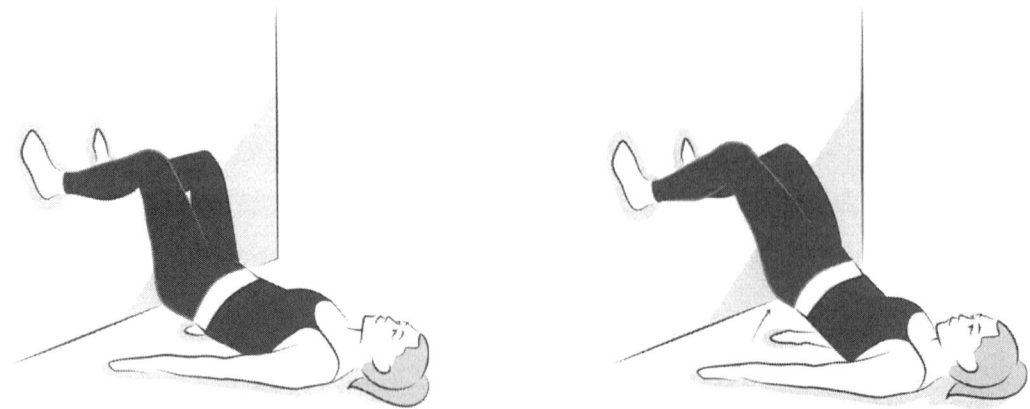

Pelvic Thrust with Wall Stability

Position yourself sitting, feet on the wall, and your hands on the floor. Initiate Pilates sequential breathing, engaging your abdomen. Inhale as you lift your pelvis upward, making a thrusting motion.

Exhale as you lower your pelvis back to the ground, promoting abdominal and leg muscle activation.

Sets and Repetitions: Perform 2 sets of 15 repetitions.

Targets: Abdominal and glute muscles.

Purpose: This exercise utilizes Pilates sequential breathing to engage the abdomen and promote stability in the pelvic region. This is important because "finishing the hips" (finishing them through to fully activate your glutes) is what helps you get the most out of your workout. This promotes muscle growth and tone in the glutes.

What to Feel: When thrusting your pelvis upward, focus on squeezing your glutes. Keep your abdominals tight. Be mindful of the activation in your abdominal and glute muscles throughout the exercise.

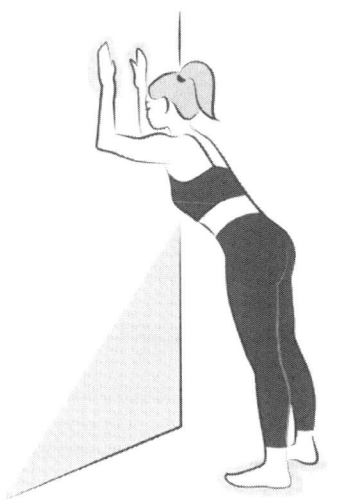 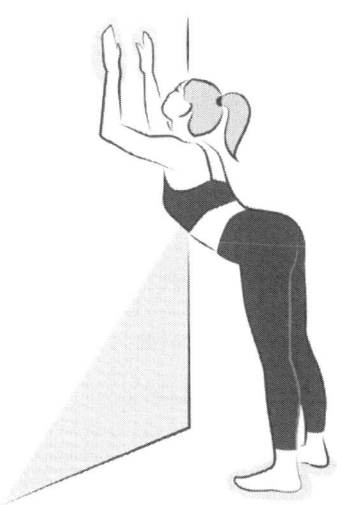

Swan Prep *(Superman Stretch)* with Wall Support

While standing, place your hands on the wall and elbows bent. Look down at the floor. Engage your abs, lifting your belly away from the wall as you inhale.

Release your spine sequentially on the exhale, returning to the starting position.

This exercise enhances back extension and strengthens core muscles.

Sets and Repetitions: Complete 3 sets of 10 repetitions.

Targets: Back extensors and core muscles.

Purpose: Enhancing back extension and core strength, this exercise focuses on controlled movements against the wall.

What to Feel: Engage your abs to lift away from the wall while inhaling, feeling the stretch in your core. During the sequential release of your spine on the exhale, focus on controlled movements and the strengthening sensation in your back extensors and core muscles.

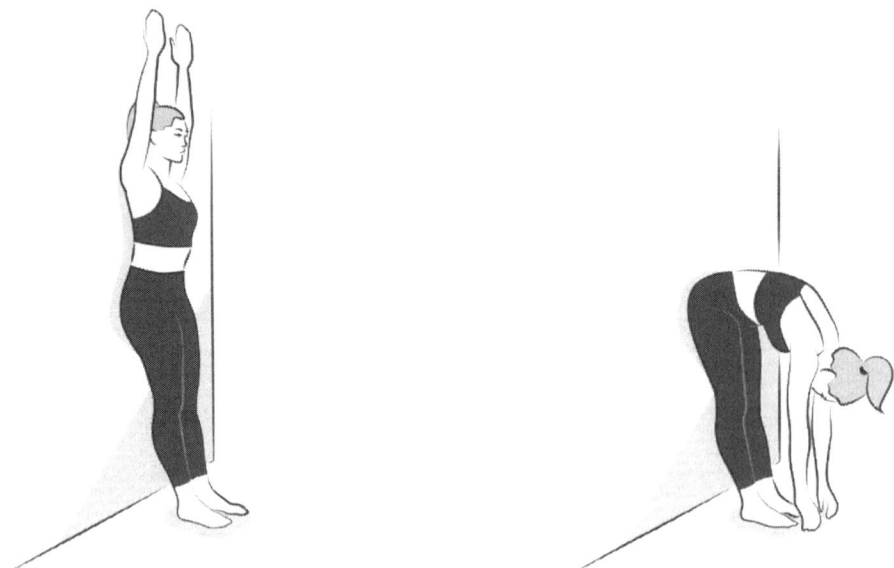

Pilates Wall Roll-Down for Abdominal Engagement

Stand with your back against the wall and feet one foot's length away. Pull your abdominal section in, raising your hands above your head. Nod your head forward, rolling your spine away from the wall while keeping abs engaged. Slowly roll down and up, feeling each vertebra touch the wall, promoting spinal articulation

Sets and Repetitions: Perform 2 sets of 8 repetitions.

Targets: Abdominal muscles and spinal articulation.

Purpose: This exercise emphasizes abdominal engagement and controlled spinal movements during the roll-down against the wall.

What to Feel: Concentrate on pulling your abdominal section in as you roll down, feeling each vertebra touch the wall. Maintain engagement throughout the movement, emphasizing the sensation of controlled abdominal activation and spinal articulation.

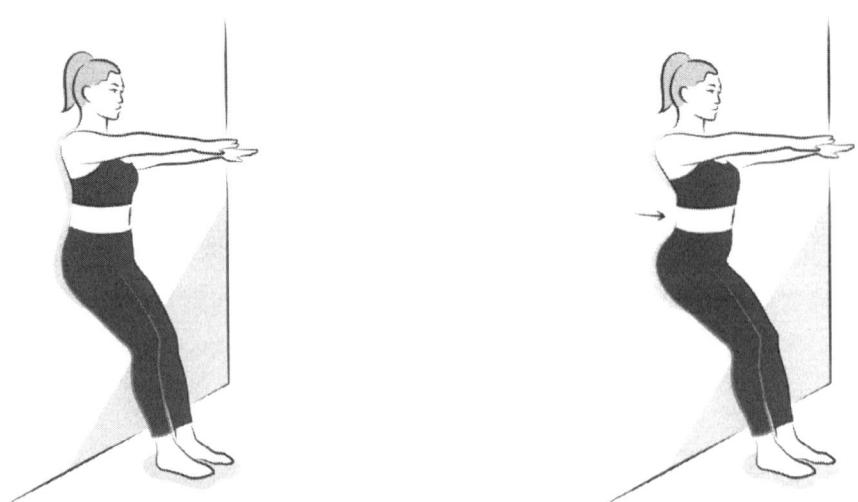

Spine Mobilization with Wall Support

Sit with your back against the wall, legs extended shoulder-width apart. Inhale, lifting your arms forward with palms facing down. Exhale, pushing your upper body forward, creating a C-shaped curve with your spine.

Use proper spinal articulation to return to the starting position, enhancing flexibility and spinal control.

Sets and Repetitions: Complete 3 sets of 10 repetitions.

Targets: Spinal flexibility and control.

Purpose: Enhancing flexibility and spinal control, this exercise involves controlled movements of the upper body against the wall.

What to Feel: Focus on the inhale, lifting your arms forward, and the exhale, pushing your upper body forward against the wall. Feel the C-shaped curve in your spine, emphasizing proper spinal articulation. Be aware of the stretch and mobility in your spine throughout the exercise.

Optimizing Recovery with Cooling Down: Unveiling the Benefits

As we diver into the realm of fitness, it's crucial not to overlook the significance of cool-down exercises, which is a phase often underestimated but laden with benefits. According to instructor Jeremy Mukhwana, cooling down is an integral part of a Wall Pilates program, serving as the concluding segment designed to promote flexibility, muscle recovery, and stress relief.

In the words of Jeremy Mukhwana, "A Wall Pilates session concludes with a cool-down period lasting about 5-10 minutes. This phase involves stretching and relaxation exercises that promote flexibility, muscle recovery, and stress relief."

Cooling down is not merely a formality; it plays a pivotal role in expediting the body's recovery process. By dedicating a few minutes to gentle stretches and relaxation techniques, individuals allow their muscles to gradually return to their resting state, reducing the likelihood of stiffness and soreness.

Beyond the immediate comfort of relieving muscle tension, the impact of cooling down reverberates in the long-term development of both muscles and metabolism. As the article suggests, incorporating cool-down exercises aids in the swift recovery of muscles, paving the way for more frequent and effective workouts. This regularity in training contributes to the gradual development and strengthening of muscles.

Furthermore, the metabolic implications of a well-structured cool-down are noteworthy. As the body cools down, it transitions from a heightened state of activity to a state of rest. This transition is essential in optimizing metabolic processes, fostering an environment where the body can efficiently utilize nutrients and energy stores.

In essence, cooling down after a Wall Pilates session becomes a holistic approach to fitness—an investment in both immediate well-being and long-term progress. By embracing the cool-down phase, individuals not only alleviate immediate post-exercise discomfort but also accelerate muscle recovery and their metabolism, propelling them toward their fitness goals with renewed vigor and efficiency.

Sample Cool-Down Exercises for Post-Wall Pilates Bliss

Cooling down is the soothing epilogue to an invigorating Wall Pilates session, and incorporating these gentle exercises into your routine ensures a harmonious transition from exertion to relaxation. Let's explore a sequence of calming cool-down exercises inspired by the BetterMe article to nurture your body and enhance recovery.

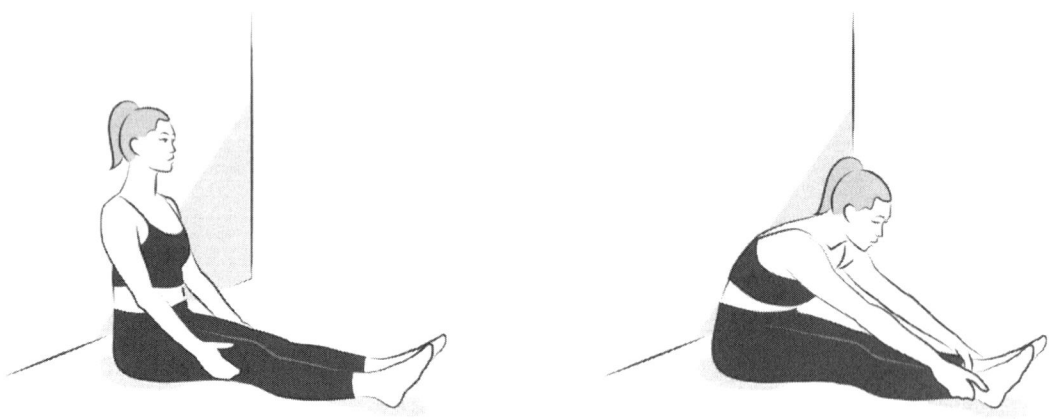

Hamstring Stretch

Sit comfortably on the floor with your legs stretched out. Inhale deeply, lengthening your spine.

Exhale as you reach forward, gently grasping your toes or shins.

Sets and Repetitions: Perform 2 sets of 15-30 seconds each.

Targets: Hamstrings.

Purpose: The purpose is to enhance flexibility in the back of the thighs. It helps alleviate tightness and promotes better range of motion.

What to Feel: Feel the stretch intensify along the back of your thighs. Concentrate on lengthening your spine during the inhale, enhancing the sensation of the stretch.

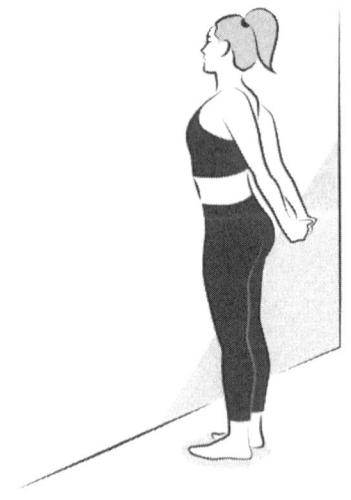

Chest Openers

Stand tall with your feet shoulder-width apart. Interlace your fingers behind your back.

Inhale, lifting your chest and squeezing your shoulder blades together.

Sets and Repetitions: Complete 3 sets, holding for 15-30 seconds.

Targets: Chest and shoulders.

Purpose: This exercise is designed to counteract the effects of slouching and sitting for extended periods. It promotes improved posture and relieves tension in the upper body.

What to Feel: Concentrate on feeling the opening and expansion across your chest.

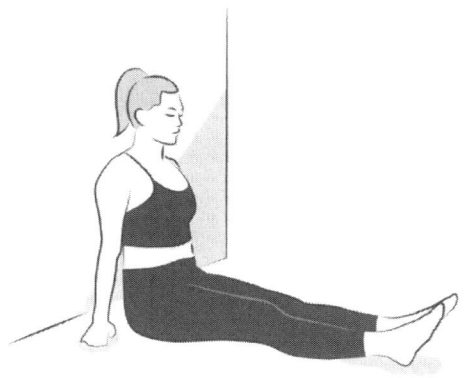 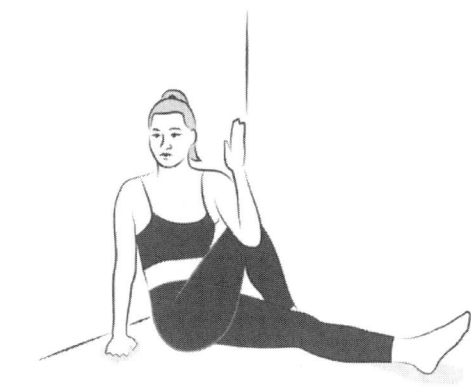

Spinal Twists

Sit cross-legged or with your legs extended. Inhale deeply, elongating your spine.

Exhale as you twist your torso to one side, placing one hand behind you and the other on your knee.

Sets and Repetitions: Perform 2 sets, holding each side for 15-30 seconds.

Targets: Spinal muscles.

Purpose: The primary purpose is to release spinal tension and improve spinal mobility. It's beneficial for those seeking relief from lower back discomfort.

What to Feel: Focus on feeling the release of tension in the spine. Pay attention to the rotational movement and the gentle release of spinal tension.

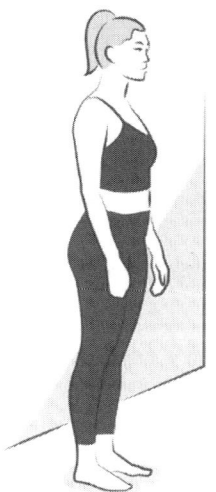 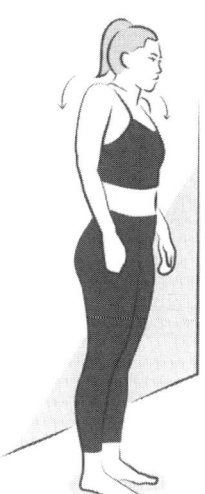

Shoulder Rolls

Stand with your feet hip-width apart.

Inhale as you lift your shoulders up toward your ears.

Exhale and roll them back and down in a circular motion.

Sets and Repetitions: Do 2 sets of 30 seconds, switching directions.

Targets: Shoulder muscles.

Purpose: This exercise aims to alleviate shoulder stiffness and tension. It promotes increased circulation and flexibility in the shoulder joints.

What to Feel: During the circular motion, focus on easing tension in the shoulders.

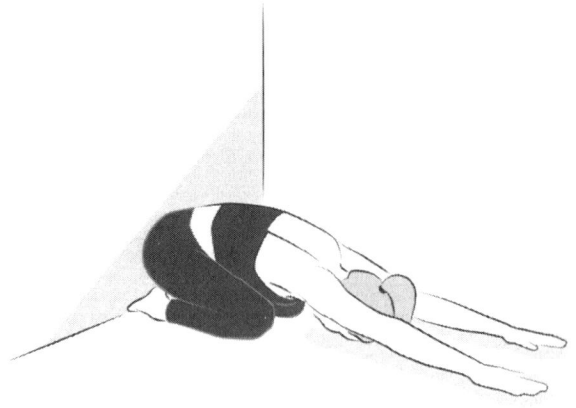

Child's Pose

Begin on your hands and knees. Sit back on your heels, reaching your arms forward. Allow your forehead to rest on the mat.

Sets and Repetitions: Perform 3 sets, holding for 30 seconds each.

Targets: Back, hips, and shoulders.

Purpose: The purpose is to stretch and release tension in the back, hips, and shoulders. It's a restorative pose that fosters relaxation and flexibility.

What to Feel: Concentrate on the sensation of relaxation and elongation in the spine.

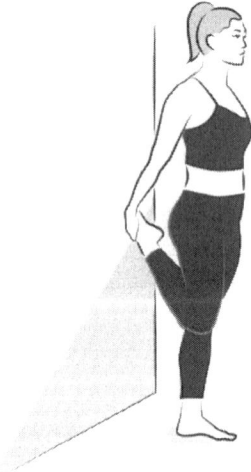

Standing Quadriceps Stretch

Stand with feet hip-width apart. Bend one knee, bringing your foot toward your buttocks.

Hold your ankle with your hand, feeling the stretch in the front of your thigh.

Sets and Repetitions: Perform 3 sets, holding for 30 seconds each.

Targets: Quadriceps.

Purpose: This exercise focuses on stretching the quadriceps muscles, promoting flexibility, and reducing tightness in the front of the thigh. It's particularly beneficial for individuals with tight hip flexors.

What to Feel: Feel the stretch in the front of your thigh.

The Interplay of Muscle Quality and Caloric Burn

Keep in mind that the relationship between muscle quality and metabolism dances in a harmonious symphony, influencing the body's ability to burn calories efficiently. This Wall Pilates program is meticulously crafted to orchestrate this metabolic symphony, sculpting not only toned and trained muscles but also fostering a lean physique that defies the conventional notion of bulkiness.

The intricacies lie in the fact that well-toned muscles serve as metabolic powerhouses, functioning as active furnaces that continuously torch calories, even in moments of repose. As the body repairs and strengthens these lean muscle fibers through targeted exercises like wall planks, squats, and leg lifts, it undergoes a transformative metamorphosis. This metamorphosis is not about cultivating bulk; rather, it's a nuanced ballet aimed at refining muscle quality.

The narrative here is clear: the more toned and trained your muscles, the swifter your metabolism becomes. This heightened metabolic rate translates into a more efficient calorie-burning mechanism, ultimately leading to decreased fat storage. Even during periods of rest or when not engaged in active exercise, these finely-tuned muscles work diligently to maintain an optimal metabolic state.

Conclusion: Nurturing the Mind-Body Synergy in Your Fitness Journey

In the pursuit of a holistic fitness journey, the connection between your mind and body is the cornerstone of your results. As we look into the significance of preparing your mind and body before a workout, the essence of mindful breathing emerged as a guiding force. While we recognize the importance of this practice, it's equally crucial to strike a balance, ensuring readers find resonance without feeling overwhelmed. The exploration of warm-up exercises provided a glimpse into the dynamic movements that prime your body for optimal workout performance, playing a pivotal role in accelerating results, fostering a robust mind-muscle connection, and laying the foundation for a results-based fitness journey.

Dynamic stretches emerged as vibrant components, infusing vitality into the warm-up routine. Transitioning into the realm of cooling down, we uncovered the pivotal role of static stretches in facilitating quicker recovery, nurturing muscles, and catalyzing metabolic development. This revelation paved the way for a deeper understanding of how muscle quality acts as a silent architect of metabolism. The more toned and trained the muscles, the more efficiently the body burns calories, even during moments of repose. This is a strategic blueprint for readers to sculpt not just a body, but a lifestyle. It's an opportunity to breathe life into the principles discussed, and works as preparation for a day of mindful movement and physical improvement with the upcoming Morning Wall Pilates Routine.

FREE BONUS:
EXERCISES CHARTS AND FULL AUDIOBOOK

I think that it can feel quite tricky to practice new exercises while holding a book open on the right page. To help with this, I have created a chart with each of the exercises pictured in this chapter enlarged and printable to make your life easier.

I have also included the full audiobook version of this book so that you can listen along as you run through your movements. I'm a big believer in giving as much as possible to each and every one of my readers to ensure that they can get the absolute most out of their exercise programs.

Go to your internet browser and type in bit.ly/wall-pilates and I'll get them to you.

You can also scan the QR Code below with your cell phone camera and tap the little link that appears if you find that easier.

All the bonuses I offer are extremely helpful and totally free!

3

MORNING WALL PILATES ROUTINE

"If you fail to prepare, you're prepared to fail."

- MARK SPITZ

Sitting on the bus, I gaze out of the window, watching the cityscape pass by in a blur. The hum of the engine creates a rhythmic backdrop to my thoughts.

Suddenly, a woman takes the seat next to me, her weary expression revealing she's had a rough start today.

"Mornings, huh? I can't stand them."

I glance at her, offering a small, polite smile.

"Why is that?" I ask.

"It's like the world's too loud too early. I always just feel so lazy and want to stay in bed."

I nod, but I can't relate.

Having been a Wall Pilates instructor for many years, I've come to start my days with a dynamic and immersive Wall Pilates routine. Doing this helps me start my day off right and inspires me for what is to come.

So, taking a deep breath, I decide to engage in a conversation with the woman about the awesome benefits of starting the day with Wall Pilates.

"You know, I used to feel the same way about mornings until I discovered something that changed my perspective," I reveal.

She looks at me with curiosity, prompting me to continue.

"Ever heard of Wall Pilates?" I ask. "It's this amazing routine that not only wakes up your body but also sets the tone for the entire day. It makes you feel productive, focused, like a high achiever."

"Wall Pilates? What's that?" the woman asks.

I explain the concept, detailing how the support of a wall adds stability, making the exercises accessible even for beginners.

"The thing about Wall Pilates is that it's not just about physical exercise. It's like a secret weapon for your mind too. The focus on concentration and control aligns with traditional Pilates principles, bringing clarity and mental sharpness."

"Huh, really?" She seems intrigued, so I decide to explain some of the ways that following the right fitness program can give you both physical and mental benefits.

"Starting the day with Wall Pilates helps you cultivate discipline and commitment. It's not just about the workout; it's a conscious choice to kickstart your day with intention. You feel more motivated, ready to tackle whatever comes your way. Trust me, it's a game-changer."

"Hmm, that sounds interesting," the woman says. "I could use some of that."

"Absolutely! It's not about hating mornings; it's about making them work for you. Wall Pilates can turn your mornings into a positive and empowering experience. Give it a shot, and you might find yourself looking forward to mornings."

As our conversation unfolds, I share more details about specific exercises, the invigorating feeling post-routine, and how it becomes a ritual of self-care. The bus ride transforms into a journey of inspiration, with the potential to reshape her mornings and mindset.

During my journey as a proponent of morning Wall Pilates, I've witnessed countless transformations in individuals just like the woman on the bus. The power of starting the day with intention, focus, and a commitment to self-improvement is truly remarkable. Many have experienced heightened productivity, a greater sense of discipline, and increased motivation throughout the day. The unique blend of physical and mental benefits that Wall Pilates offers contributes not only to improved strength, flexibility, and posture but also to a positive mindset that resonates beyond the workout. It's more than a fitness routine; it's a holistic approach to well-being, and I've seen individuals embrace their days with newfound energy, positivity, and a high-achiever mindset, all stemming from the simple but effective practice of morning Wall Pilates.

The Transformative Power of Morning Wall Pilates for Body and Mind

Beginning each day with a morning Wall Pilates routine massively benefits both the body and the mind. Drawing insights from articles by Pilates instructors Liz McKee and Julie Carolan, the advantages become evident. Wall Pilates, with its unique combination of traditional Pilates principles and the support of a wall, offers a holistic approach to fitness.

Physically, engaging in Wall Pilates in the morning serves as an invigorating wake-up call for the body. As noted by Liz McKee's article, "10 Top Tips for Your Morning Pilates Routine", this innovative program addresses common imbalances caused by sedentary lifestyles, activating underused muscles, enhancing body awareness, and incorporating functional training. The use of the wall as a support system provides stability, allowing individuals to maintain balance and proper alignment, particularly beneficial for beginners or those with balance issues.

In her article, "Benefits of Morning Pilates", Julie Carolan emphasizes the importance of morning Pilates in preparing the body for the day. The slow-paced, whole-body workout ensures correct muscle engagement, good posture, and endurance. As the body gradually wakes up, Wall Pilates incorporates stretching, breathwork, and strengthening exercises, effectively loosening out the body and priming it to take on daily challenges.

The benefits extend beyond the physical realm, influencing the reader's mental state and overall well-being. Morning exercise, as highlighted by Julie Carolan, positively impacts mood by releasing endorphins, fostering a sense of accomplishment that lasts throughout the day. Wall Pilates, with its focus on concentration, control, and flow, aligns with the principles of traditional Pilates, contributing to improved mental focus and clarity.

Setting up the day for productivity and achievement, engaging in morning Wall Pilates can enhance the reader's sense of discipline and commitment to their fitness goals. McKee emphasizes the importance of consistency and patience in seeing improvements in strength, flexibility, and posture. The routine becomes a ritual, a mindful practice that aligns with the reader's overarching goals.

Incorporating Wall Pilates into the morning routine is not just a physical exercise; it's a deliberate choice to start the day with intention. The unique blend of stability, resistance, and versatility offered by Wall Pilates positions individuals to approach their day with a sense of purpose, focus, and motivation. As the body becomes toned, strong, flexible, and lean, you will not only experience physical transformation but also set the tone for a day of high achievement and fulfillment.

In essence, the practice of morning Wall Pilates becomes a ritual of self-care, a gateway to physical and mental well-being that resonates throughout the day. The reader emerges from this routine not only physically energized but also mentally prepared to tackle challenges, stay focused on their goals, and embrace the day with a high-achiever mindset.

A Dynamic Morning Wall Pilates Routine

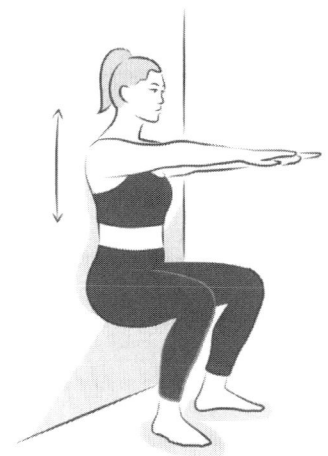

Exercise 1: Wall Squats

Stand with back against the wall, feet hip-width apart. Slide down into a squat position, knees aligned with ankles.

Press through heels to return to the starting position.

Sets and Repetitions: Perform 3 sets of 15 repetitions.

Targets: Targets the quadriceps, hamstrings, and glutes.

Purpose: The purpose is to strengthen the lower body muscles and improve squat form with the support of the wall.

What to Feel: Focus on maintaining proper squat form, ensuring the knees align with the ankles. Feel the engagement in your quads and glutes as you press through the heels to return to the starting position.

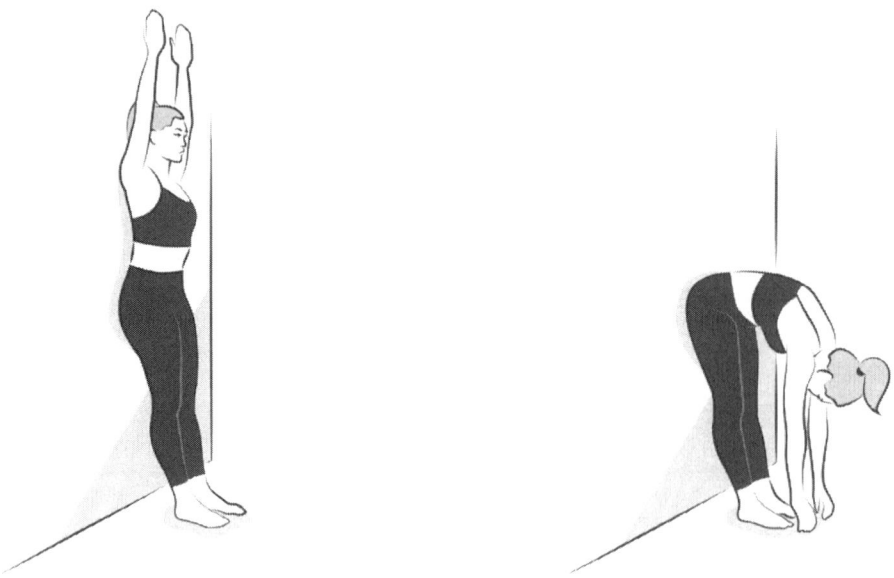

Exercise 2: Wall Roll Down

Face away from the wall, using it for support if needed, with feet hip-width apart. Slowly hinge at your hips and roll your upper body downward, reaching your hands to the floor. Roll back up, stacking each vertebra for improved flexibility.

Sets and Repetitions: Do 2 sets of 10 repetitions.

Targets: Spine mobility, hamstrings, and core.

Purpose: The purpose is to enhance flexibility in the spine and hamstrings while also engaging the core during the roll-down and roll-up motions.

What to Feel: Focus on a slow and controlled descent towards the floor, reaching your hands to touch the wall. Feel each vertebra stacking as you roll back up, emphasizing improved flexibility in the spine.

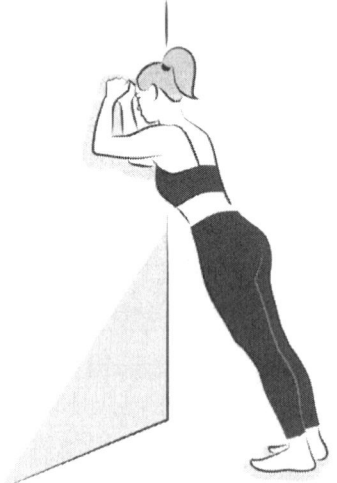

Exercise 3: Wall Plank

Place your forearms on the wall, with elbows at shoulder height.

Step back into a plank position, maintaining a straight line from head to heels, draw your belly button inward and hold to engage your core muscles.

Sets and Repetitions: Perform 3 sets, holding for 30 seconds each.

Targets: The core, shoulders, and arms.

Purpose: The purpose is to build strength and stability in the core, shoulders, and arms in a plank position against the wall.

What to Feel: Focus on maintaining a straight line from head to heels. Feel the engagement in your core, shoulders, and arms as you hold the plank position.

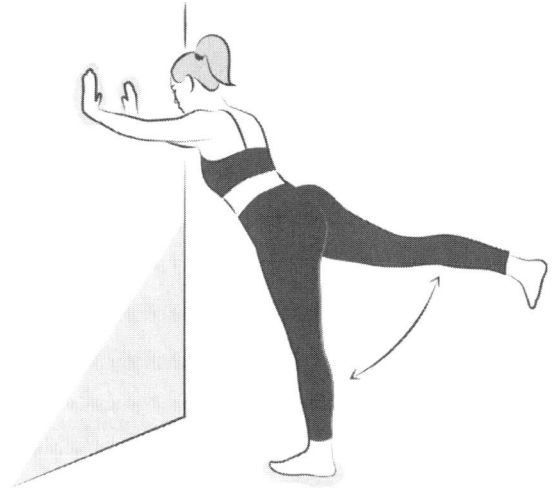

Exercise 4: Wall Leg Lifts

Stand facing the wall with your hands against it for support.

Lift one leg straight back to fully engage your glutes and hamstrings.

Lower the leg and switch to the other. Control each leg-lift to fully target the lower body.

Sets and Repetitions: Do 3 sets of 12 repetitions per leg.

Targets: Glutes, hamstrings, and lower body.

Purpose: The purpose is to strengthen and tone the lower body muscles with controlled leg lifts.

What to Feel: Focus on engaging your glutes and hamstrings as you lift one leg straight back. Feel the controlled movement and switch legs to target the entire lower body.

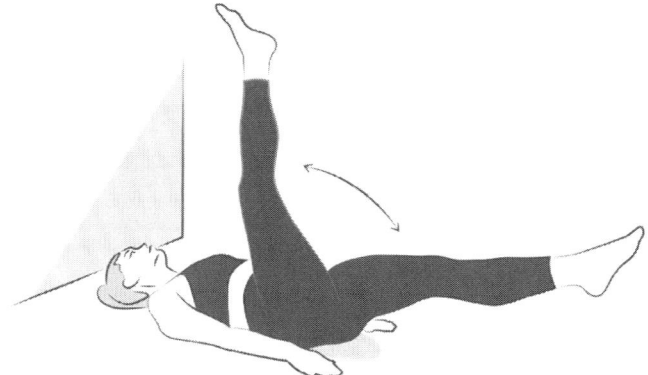

Exercise 5: Scissor Kicks

Lie on your back, hands pressed into the floor.

Lift legs vertically and scissor them in controlled movements.

Sets and Repetitions: Perform 2 sets of 20 scissor kicks.

Targets: The core and lower abdominal muscles.

Purpose: The purpose is to challenge the core with dynamic leg movements while lying on your back.

What to Feel: Focus on pressing your hands into the floor for stability and feel the engagement in your core as you scissor kick your legs vertically.

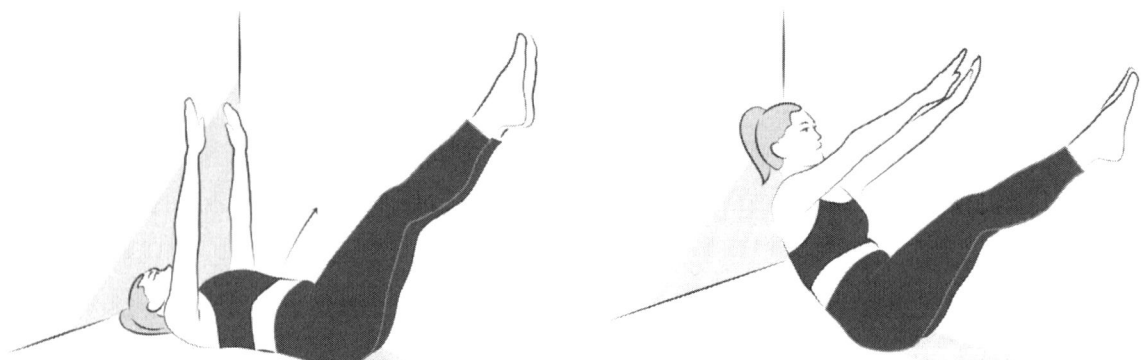

Exercise 6: Core Teasers

Start by lying flat on your back. Lift your straight legs off the ground.

Extend your arm toward your feet, engage your abs, and roll your body up halfway, then roll back down.

Sets and Repetitions: Do 3 sets of 12 teasers.

Targets: The core, balance, and coordination.

Purpose: The purpose is to enhance core strength and improve balance and coordination with the rolling motion against the wall.

What to Feel: Focus on lifting your legs into a tabletop position, rolling down halfway, and then rolling back up. Feel the challenge in your core throughout the movement.

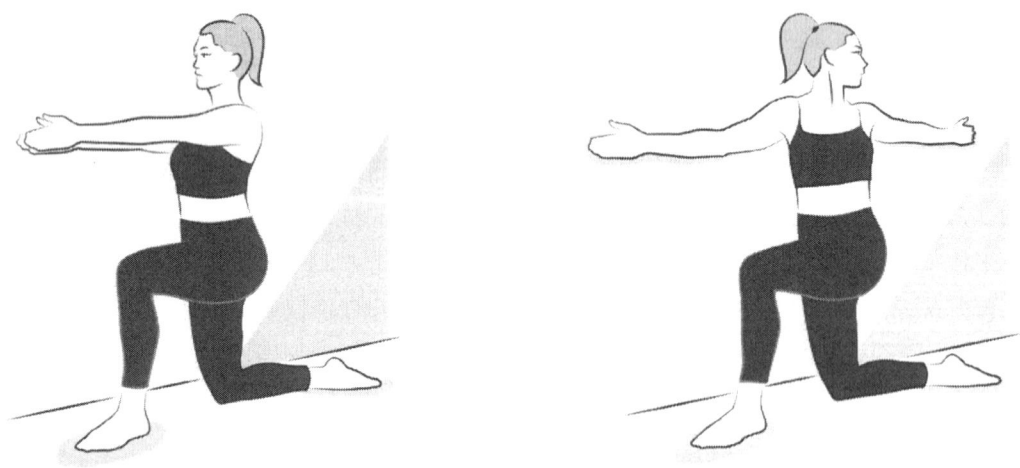

Exercise 7: Wall Rotation

In a lunge position with your knee closest to the wall on the floor and both arms extended in front (palms together). Rotate your torso and separate your arms, expanding your chest, until both arms are touching the wall. Return to the start position under control.

Sets and Repetitions: Perform 2 sets of 15 rotations on each side.

Targets: The obliques and improves spinal mobility.

Purpose: The purpose is to strengthen the oblique muscles and enhance flexibility in the spine with controlled rotations against the wall.

What to Feel: Focus on keeping your back against the wall while rotating your torso from side to side. Feel the engagement in your obliques.

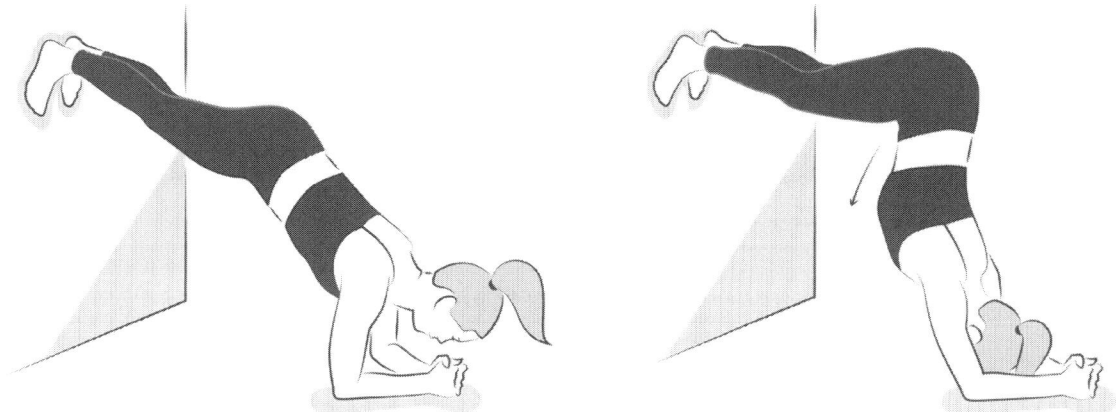

Exercise 8: Wall Pike

Assume a plank position with feet on the wall. Lift hips towards the ceiling, forming an inverted V shape.

Sets and Repetitions: Do 3 sets of 12 pikes.

Targets: The core and enhances flexibility.

Purpose: The purpose is to build core strength and flexibility with the challenging pike movement in a plank position with feet on the wall.

What to Feel: Focus on lifting your hips towards the ceiling, forming an inverted V shape. Feel the intense engagement in your core throughout the movement.

As we conclude this exploration of the Morning Wall Pilates routine, it's evident that this practice goes beyond physical exercise; it's a holistic approach to starting the day with purpose and vitality. By embracing stability, resistance, and versatility, individuals not only sculpt their bodies but also cultivate a mindset of focus and achievement. The benefits resonate throughout the day, fostering a sense of discipline and motivation.

Now, let's seamlessly transition into the next chapter, and discover the equally rewarding realm of Evening Wall Pilates. This routine offers a unique perspective on unwinding, reenergizing, and promoting relaxation after a day's challenges, ensuring a balanced and holistic approach to well-being.

FREE BONUS:
EXERCISE VIDEOS GUIDES

To make sure that you get the most out of every single one of your workouts, I have included video guides that demonstrate every exercise, movement, and brace that a part of this book. These reference videos have been put together so that you can visualize and understand each movement, and then apply the written teaching points that the book provides to ensure that you fully engage your target muscles, and so that you can maintain excellent form while doing so.

Go to your internet browser and type in bit.ly/wall-pilates and I'll get them over to you right away.

You can also scan the QR Code below with your cell phone camera and tap the little link that appears if you find that easier.

All the bonuses I offer are extremely helpful and totally free!

4

EVENING WALL PILATES ROUTINE

"Nothing is impossible. The word itself says I'm Possible."
- AUDREY HEPBURN

As I walk into my niece's birthday party, the joyful chatter and excitement surround me. My sister, holding the elaborately decorated cake, greets me with a smile.

But then, disaster strikes.

Just as we're about to sing "Happy Birthday," my sister lets out a loud yawn and in turn, trips over her own feet.

"Woah," she cries out as this mistake threatens to turn the cake-cutting into a disaster.

I instinctively reach out and steady the cake, averting a potential catastrophe.

Phew.

Amid the collective sighs of relief, my sister chuckles nervously, "I really need to get more sleep; I've been so clumsy lately."

I frown, because I know what it's like to struggle with getting enough sleep at night.

Even now, in a time where I've managed to find balance, my mind often drifts back to those teenage years when sleep was elusive, and each night became a battleground of tossing and turning. The relentless struggle to find solace in the embrace of slumber left me fatigued and lethargic the next day. The weight of sleepless nights became a heavy burden, impacting my energy, focus, and overall well-being.

It's a distant memory now, but the echoes of those restless nights serve as a poignant reminder of the importance of a good night's sleep for both physical and mental vitality.

Now, as I reflect on those years, I find solace in the power of Wall Pilates, a practice that has become an integral part of my nighttime routine. Incorporating these gentle yet effective exercises into my evenings has changed my life for the better. The targeted stretches and mindful movements help alleviate back pain, release the tension accumulated throughout the day, and provide a sanctuary to let go of the stresses that linger. It's not just a physical practice; it's a ritual of bringing my body back into balance, preparing it for a restorative night's sleep. The soothing embrace of Wall Pilates has become my ally in the journey to peaceful nights and energized mornings.

Concerned, I reply to my sister, "You know, I've found that doing Wall Pilates in the evening has helped me relax and sleep better. Maybe it could work for you too?"

My sister looks unsure as we sit down to catch our breath after the cake-saving moment.

"You really think so?"

"Yes!" I begin, "there was a time when I couldn't sleep well at all. Tossing and turning, restless nights, you name it. But then I discovered Wall Pilates, and it transformed my evenings." My sister looks intrigued, so I continue, "Incorporating it into my nightly routine helped reduce my back pain, release tension, and create a sense of balance. I found myself letting go of the day's stress and sleeping like a baby. It's been a game-changer for me, and I thought you might find it beneficial too."

As we continue our conversation, and the party buzzes around us, the focus shifts to the potential of Wall Pilates to bring a peaceful night's sleep.

In a world where many people, including myself and my sister, grapple with the challenge of falling asleep, the introduction of Wall Pilates into the evening routine emerges as a promising solution. The soothing exercises not only alleviate the struggles of insomnia but also bring a myriad of additional benefits. From reducing back pain to releasing accumulated tension, Wall Pilates becomes a holistic approach to enhancing overall well-being. As the awareness of these transformative effects spreads, more individuals are discovering the potential of this practice to not only nurture physical health but also to foster a peaceful and restful night's sleep.

Evening Harmony: Unwinding with Wall Pilates

Finishing an active day with an evening Wall Pilates routine offers a holistic approach to nurturing both the body and the mind. As highlighted in Marchel Ackler's article, "What is Wall Pilates?", the benefits of this practice extend beyond the physical realm, delving into the realms of relaxation, stress relief, and overall well-being. Ackler notes, "Wall Pilates can also help with menstrual cramps as it lengthens and opens the lower back muscles and pelvis, which can help with pain relief." This underlines the tangible physical benefits, providing a soothing solution for discomfort and tension. Moreover, the article emphasizes the positive impact on sleep, stating, "Wall Pilates and Pilates in general can help you get a better night's sleep. A combination of the stress relief provided by this workout and deep breathing exercises will improve how much and how well you sleep." Engaging in Wall Pilates during the evening becomes a mindful ritual, creating a dedicated space for individuals to unwind, release the stresses of the day, and bring their bodies back into balance.

In the realm of mindfulness and mental well-being, the evening Wall Pilates routine plays a crucial role. By incorporating this practice into their evenings, individuals can tap into the power of mindfulness to stay motivated and cultivate happiness. The intentional and controlled movements in Wall Pilates encourage participants to focus on the present moment, fostering a sense of mindfulness that transcends the physical aspects of the workout. This mindful practice becomes a sanctuary for letting go of daily stressors, promoting mental clarity, and cultivating a positive mindset.

As the body engages in the gentle yet effective exercises, the mind follows suit, finding solace and tranquility in the rhythmic flow of the routine. Beyond the physical benefits of reduced back pain and improved sleep, Wall Pilates becomes a conduit for mental rejuvenation. The deliberate choice to prioritize self-care in the evening through Wall Pilates sets the stage for a restful night's sleep and contributes to waking up the next day with a refreshed body and a motivated, happier mindset. In essence, the evening Wall Pilates routine becomes a holistic practice that nurtures the intricate connection between physical and mental well-being, creating a harmonious balance in one's life.

An Evening Wall Pilates Routine

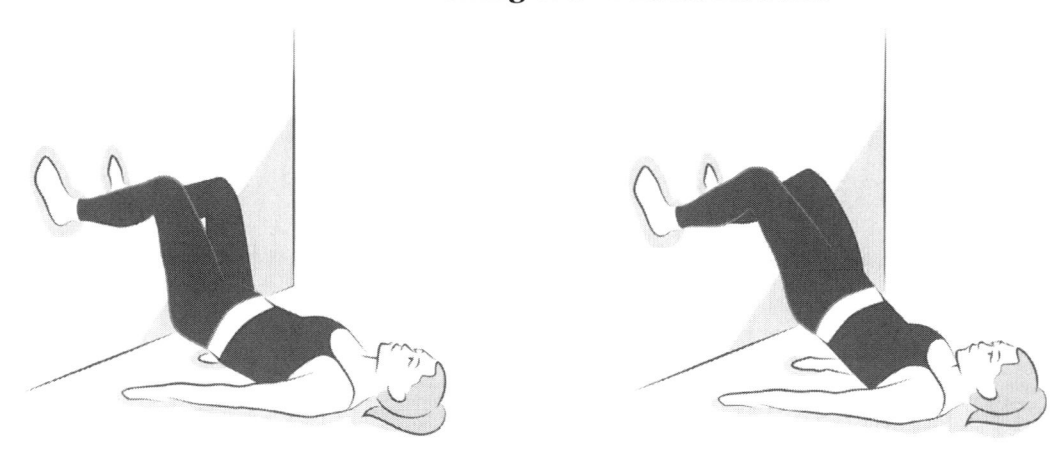

Exercise 1: Wall Bridge

Lie on your back with feet against the wall, knees bent. Lift hips towards the ceiling, so that your shoulders, hips and knees are in a straight line.

Sets and Repetitions: Do 3 sets of 12 repetitions.

Targets: Glutes, hamstrings, and lower back.

Purpose: The purpose is to activate and strengthen the glutes and hamstrings, promoting lower body stability.

What to Feel: Focus on lifting your hips towards the ceiling to create a straight line from shoulders to knees. Feel the contraction in your glutes and hamstrings during the bridge movement.

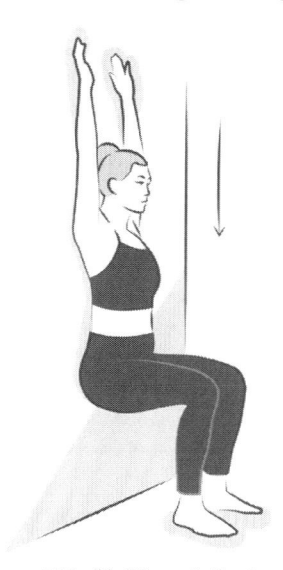

Exercise 2: Wall Sit with Arm Raises

Stand against the wall, lower into a seated position. Hold your arms straight out, then raise overhead.

Sets and Repetitions: Perform 2 sets of 20 seconds each.

Targets: Quadriceps, shoulders, and arms.

Purpose: The purpose is to engage the lower body in a seated position against the wall while incorporating arm raises for added shoulder engagement.

What to Feel: Focus on holding the seated position against the wall. Feel the burn in your quadriceps and the engagement in your shoulders as you raise your arms overhead.

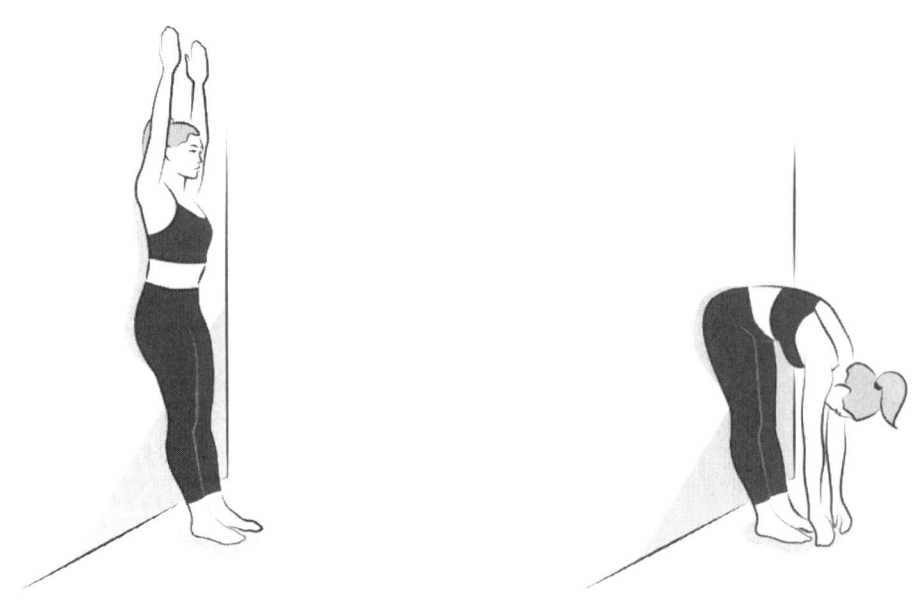

Exercise 3: Wall Roll-Downs

Face away from the wall, using it for support if needed, with feet hip-width apart. Slowly roll the spine down, reaching towards the floor. Roll back up, engaging core.

Sets and Repetitions: Perform 3 sets of 10 repetitions.

Targets: Back, spinal erectors, arms and shoulders.

Purpose: The purpose of this exercise is to improve flexibility and mobility in the spine, strengthen the muscles in the back, and engage the core for overall stability. It also helps enhance body awareness and posture.

What to Feel: Focus on a gentle stretch along the spine as you roll down towards the floor. You should feel a lengthening sensation in the muscles of your back. As you roll back up, engage your core muscles to support the spine and feel a contraction in your abdominal area. Ensure a controlled and deliberate motion throughout the exercise to maximize its benefits.

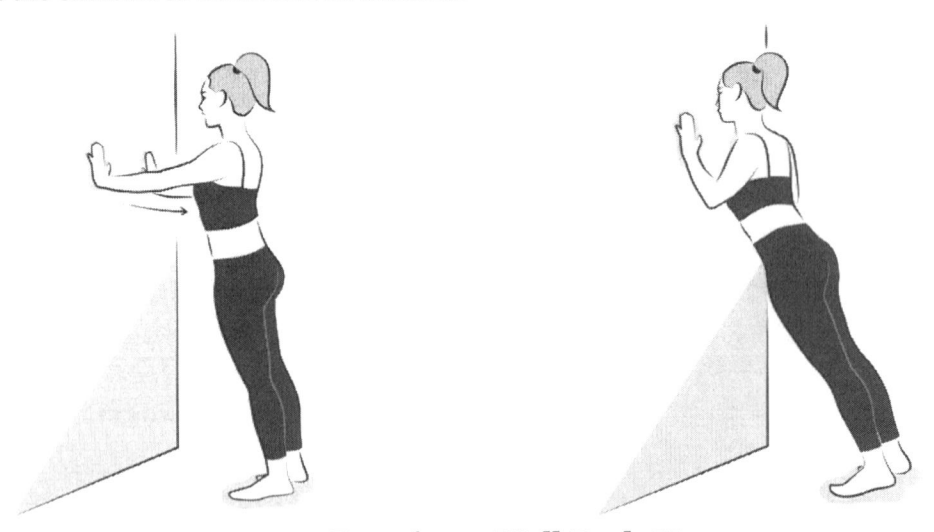

Exercise 4: Wall Push-Ups

Stand arm's length away from the wall, with your hands a little wider than shoulders width apart, and your body weight braced and leaning forwards. Aim your chest between your hands, feeling your chest and arm muscles engage and stretch as you lower yourself toward the wall. Push your body back to the start position, driving up through your chest, while keeping a strong posture.

Sets and Repetitions: Perform 3 sets of 12 repetitions.

Targets: Chest, triceps, and shoulders.

Purpose: The purpose is to strengthen the upper body through a modified push-up against the wall.

What to Feel: Aim your chest between your hands, feeling your chest and arm muscles engage and stretch. Lift your chest upward, ensuring a sturdy and upright posture.

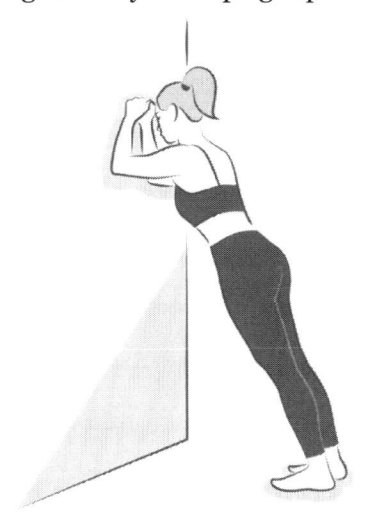

Exercise 5: Wall Plank

Face the wall, hands on it, step feet back to a plank.

Sets and Repetitions: Perform 3 sets, bracing for 30-45 seconds for each.

Targets: The core, shoulders, and arms.

Purpose: The purpose is to build strength and stability in the core, shoulders, and arms in a plank position against the wall.

What to Feel: Focus on maintaining a straight line from head to heels. Feel the engagement in your core, shoulders, and arms as you hold the plank position.

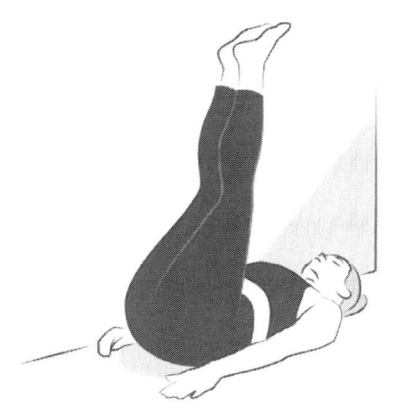

Exercise 6: Legs Up the Wall Stretch

Sit in an L-shaped position against the wall. Swing your legs up so that the hips are in a flexed position, and they rest against the wall (in this case the side of the right leg).

Hold the position for 30 seconds, feeling a gentle stretch in your hamstrings and lower back. Lower your legs and rest for 10 seconds.

Sets and Repetitions: Hold for 2 minutes.

Targets: Hamstrings, lower back, and promotes relaxation.

Purpose: The purpose is to stretch and release tension in the hamstrings and lower back while promoting relaxation.

What to Feel: Focus on swinging your legs up the wall and feel the gentle stretch along your hamstrings and lower back. Allow yourself to relax into the stretch.

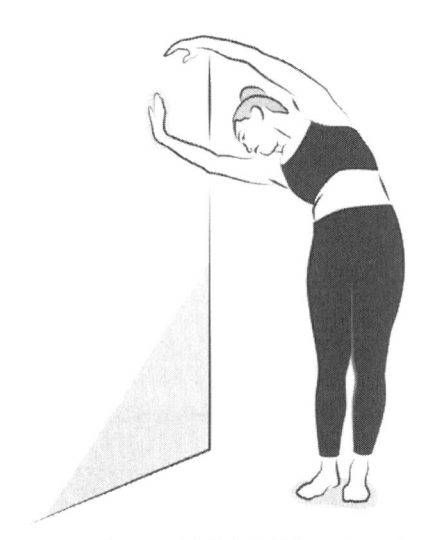

Exercise 7: Wall Side Bend

Stand with your side facing the wall, raise your arm overhead. Lean towards the wall.

Sets and Repetitions: Perform 2 sets of 12 repetitions on each side.

Targets: Targets the obliques and lateral muscles.

Purpose: The purpose is to strengthen the oblique muscles and improve lateral flexibility.

What to Feel: Focus on raising your arm overhead and leaning towards the wall, feeling the stretch along your side. Emphasize the engagement in your obliques.

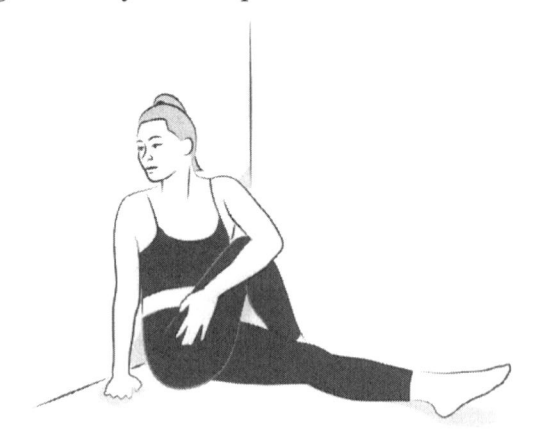

Exercise 8: Seated Wall Twist

Sit with your back against the wall, cross your right leg over left.

Doing this will make you feel less tense, as it enhances flexibility and mobility. It engages your oblique muscles, making you feel a gentle contraction.

Sets and Repetitions: Do 3 sets of 10 repetitions per side.

Targets: The obliques and promotes spinal mobility.

Purpose: The purpose is to enhance spinal mobility and strengthen the oblique muscles through twisting movements.

What to Feel: Feel less tension as it enhances flexibility and mobility. Focus on the gentle contraction of your oblique muscles during the twist, promoting a sense of release and flexibility.

As we enter the realm of Pilates routines, the transition from the calming embrace of evening Wall Pilates to the efficiency of a 15-minute Wall Pilates routine marks a shift in focus. While the evening routines aim to unwind and relax, the condensed 15-minute sessions are designed for those seeking a quick yet effective burst of Pilates. In the upcoming exploration, we'll uncover the art of maximizing benefits in a limited timeframe.

These concise routines offer an accessible entry point for those with busy schedules, ensuring that the advantages of Wall Pilates can be integrated into even the busiest person's daily life. Join me as I unravel the potency of these time-efficient sessions, providing a pathway for individuals to prioritize their well-being without compromising on time.

FREE BONUS:
WALL PILATES PICTURE CHARTS

I have put together each of the pictured Wall Pilates exercises from this chapter into easy-to-follow picture charts that you can print out to use alongside the video guides and book descriptions to ensure that you can maximize the effectiveness of your workouts.

To access these, go to your internet browser and type in bit.ly/wall-pilates and I'll email them to you.

You can also scan the QR Code below with your cell phone camera and tap the little link that appears if you find that easier.

All the bonuses I offer are extremely helpful and totally free!

5

15-MINUTE WALL PILATES ROUTINES

"Exercise is medicine. It should be prescribed by your doctor and only taken regularly in the dose that works for you."

- BOB HARPER

"I wish I had slimmer and more toned abs! Why is that so hard to get?"

I'm standing in front of the dressing room mirror, eyeing a bold red dress that caught my attention. The store's lighting is subtle, creating a tranquil atmosphere amid the faint rustling of clothes and hushed whispers. As I consider trying on the dress, snippets of conversation from the adjacent changing stall capture my attention.

A woman's voice drifts through the thin walls, discussing her fitness goals with a friend.

"And a bigger booty would be nice. Plus, I'd love to have leaner arms... you know, no more 'triceps' jiggle." Her frustration is palpable as she adds, "But with work and everything, I just don't have the time to hit the gym."

Her words resonate with the societal pressures we often face regarding body image. I find myself empathizing with her struggles, the desire for a certain physique conflicting with the demands of a hectic life.

"Back fat," she mentions, the phrase hanging in the air. "I hate it!"

It's a raw moment, a glimpse into the universal challenge of striving for physical perfection while navigating a packed schedule.

Taking a deep breath, I consider the importance of self-love and acceptance in this journey towards wellness. It's a reminder that each person's path is unique, and understanding and compassion should be at the forefront.

Yet... as I stand there, contemplating the empowering notion of feeling good in one's own skin, I feel a surge of inspiration. It's as if the universe is nudging me to share something positive with the woman in the neighboring stall.

Taking a deep breath, I decide to help this woman out.

With a determined stride, I head towards the curtain that separates us.

"Excuse me," I say gently, "I couldn't help but overhear your conversation. I wanted to share something that might resonate with your goals."

The woman turns, her eyes curious but guarded.

I start explaining the benefits of Wall Pilates, highlighting its efficiency in achieving fitness goals on a tight schedule.

"It's a fantastic way to work on your abs, tone your arms, and even engage those glutes," I share with a warm smile. "And the best part? Some programs are so quick, you will be done in just fifteen minutes."

As we continue our conversation, the atmosphere shifts from a dressing room to a shared space of understanding. I share how wall Pilates has been a game-changer for many, fitting seamlessly into busy schedules. The woman, initially skeptical, begins to express genuine interest.

In the midst of the clothing racks and hushed whispers, we discuss the simplicity of these exercises and the positive impact they can have on both body and mind, even in a time crunch.

It becomes more than a conversation about fitness; it transforms into a dialogue about embracing one's journey with self-love and discovering achievable ways to prioritize well-being.

"You know what?" the woman says. "You are right. It's important to have a short and sharp workout on hand... I can actually fit that into my schedule!"

I smile. "That's right. It's all about finding a way that works within the time you have available, and then booking it into your schedule, just like you would with any other appointment."

Feeling satisfied with the conversation, I turn away.

When that red dress catches my eye again, I don't hesitate. Feeling invigorated and empowered, I snatch it off the rack and head toward the cashier.

Juggling Life, Sculpting Dreams:
A Universal Struggle for Fitness and Well-Being

In a world where women juggle myriad responsibilities, the desire to look and feel good often takes a backseat to the demands of daily life. The woman in the dressing store, expressing her longing for slimmer abs, a toned booty, and leaner arms while lamenting the time constraints, is not alone. Many of us share these aspirations, yet finding the time for lengthy workout routines seems elusive.

The truth is this struggle is universal. The societal expectations and standards for beauty can create a constant undercurrent of pressure. But amidst the chaos, there's a silver lining... a solution that caters to the busy lifestyles we lead. Wall Pilates emerges as a beacon of hope, offering quick and effective workouts that can be seamlessly woven into any schedule.

Finding time for oneself can be a formidable challenge. Joanne Sutton, a devoted carer for her mother dealing with health issues, understands this struggle intimately in her article, "How Do You Fit Pilates Into Your Tight Schedule?" Reflecting on her own experiences, she shares creative ways to incorporate Pilates into a busy schedule, emphasizing the importance of self-care to prevent burnout.

Joanne advocates for the flexibility of Pilates sessions, suggesting that being open to variable session times is key. She acknowledges personal preferences but highlights the significance of adapting to unpredictable schedules. Joanne's approach is a testament to her commitment to self-care, stating, "Sometimes it's in the afternoon and other times it's the evening depending on when my Mum is taking a nap or is asleep for the night."

The beauty of wall Pilates lies in its accessibility. It doesn't demand a dedicated hour at the gym or a complex workout space. Instead, it adapts to the nooks and crannies of our lives. Whether at home, in the office, or even during a break at the park, wall Pilates proves to be a versatile companion.

Drawing inspiration from James Clear's "Atomic Habits," Joanne explores the concept of habit stacking to establish a consistent Pilates practice. By attaching new habits to existing ones, she creates neural connections that make maintaining these habits more achievable. Joanne shares her personal example of stacking balance training onto her foot routine, showcasing how small, intentional additions can lead to significant results.

The quick, 15-minute routines become a game-changer. Tailored to engage muscles from head to toe, these workouts address the very areas that the dressing store woman and countless others wish to tone and sculpt. The wall becomes a multifunctional piece of equipment, transforming any space into a personal fitness haven.

What sets Wall Pilates apart is its flexibility, both in terms of time and location. It dismantles the notion that achieving fitness goals requires lengthy, rigorous sessions. Now, every woman can take charge of her well-being without sacrificing precious time.

As we collectively navigate the complexities of modern life, wall Pilates stands as an ally... a reminder that self-care is a necessity, not a luxury. It's a call to embrace the journey towards feeling good in our own skin, acknowledging that small, consistent efforts are what lead to significant transformations. So, to every woman yearning for a fitness solution that aligns with her bustling lifestyle, Wall Pilates beckons... an invitation to prioritize herself, anytime, anywhere.

Beginner Wall Pilates Routines (15 minutes or less)

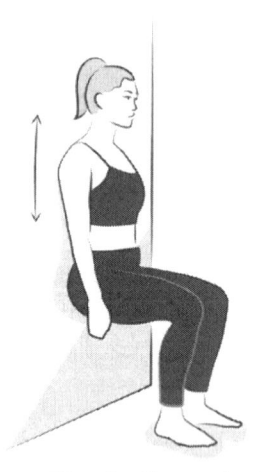

Exercise 1: Basic Core Activation

Stand with your back against the wall. Engage your core and slowly slide down the wall into a seated position.

Hold the seated position for up to 30 seconds, focus on drawing your abs in while gently pressing your lower back towards the wall to maintain core engagement.

Slide back up the wall to the starting position.

Sets and Repetitions: 3 sets of 10 repetitions (seated to standing).

Targets: Core muscles, especially the abdominal muscles.

Purpose: Activate and strengthen the core muscles. Improve overall core stability.

What to Feel: Focus on maintaining core engagement throughout the movement. Feel the activation in your abdominal muscles. Pay attention to the smooth transition between seated and standing positions.

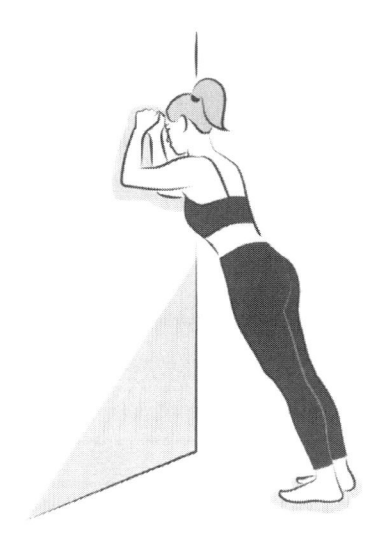

Exercise 2: Wall Plank

Face the wall and place your hands on it, shoulder-width apart. Step your feet back, creating a straight line from head to heels.

Hold the plank position for 40 seconds, engaging your core and glutes. Rest for 20 seconds.

Sets and Repetitions: 4 sets of 30 seconds hold, with 20 seconds rest between sets.

Targets: Core muscles, shoulders, and overall body stability.

Purpose: Develop core strength and stability. Improve shoulder strength and endurance.

What to Feel: Concentrate on engaging your core throughout the plank. Feel the tension in your shoulders and abs. Ensure a straight line from head to heels.

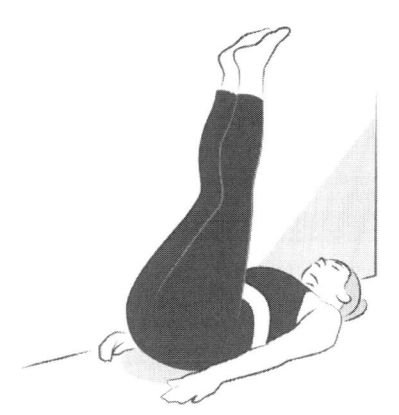

Exercise 3: Legs Up the Wall Stretch

Sit sideways next to the wall and swing your legs up, resting them against the wall. Extend your arms to the sides for balance. Hold the position for 30 seconds, feeling a gentle stretch in your hamstrings and lower back. Lower your legs and rest for 10 seconds.

Sets and Repetitions: 3 sets of 30 seconds each.

Targets: Hamstrings, lower back, and promotes flexibility.

Purpose: Stretch and relax the hamstrings and lower back. Improve flexibility in the legs.

What to Feel: Feel a gentle stretch in the hamstrings and lower back. Focus on controlled movements when lowering the legs.

Intermediate Wall Pilates Routines (15 minutes or less)

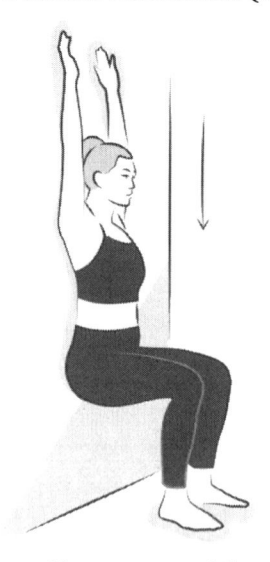

Exercise 1: Wall Squats with Arm Raises

Stand with your back against the wall. Lower into a squat position while simultaneously raising your arms overhead. Hold for 30 seconds, then return to the starting position. Rest for 15 seconds.

Sets and Repetitions: 4 sets of 12 repetitions.

Targets: Quadriceps, glutes, shoulders, and arms.

Purpose: Strengthen lower body muscles. Engage the shoulder and arm muscles. Enhance overall muscle coordination.

What to Feel: Feel the engagement in your quadriceps and glutes during the squat. Focus on raising your arms overhead to activate shoulder muscles. Maintain a stable and controlled movement.

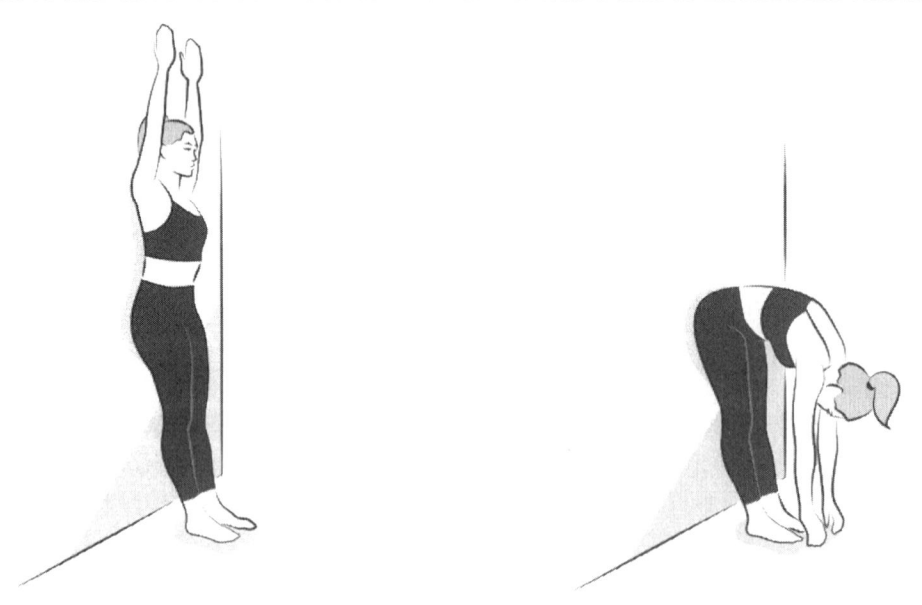

Exercise 2: Wall Roll-Downs

Stand facing the wall with arms extended. Slowly roll the spine down, reaching towards the floor. Roll back up, engaging your core.

Sets and Repetitions: 3 sets of 10 repetitions.

Targets: Spinal mobility, especially the core muscles.

Purpose: Improve flexibility and mobility of the spine. Strengthen core muscles. Enhance body awareness.

What to Feel: Feel a sequential articulation of the spine as you roll down and up. Engage your core throughout the movement. Focus on controlled and deliberate motions.

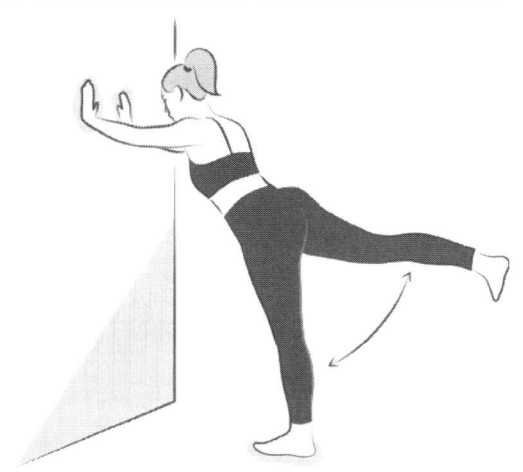

Exercise 3: Wall Plank with Leg Lifts

Start in a wall plank position. Lift one leg off the wall, keeping it straight. Hold for 20 seconds, then switch legs.

Sets and Repetitions: 5 sets of 10 leg lifts (alternating legs).

Targets: Core muscles, especially the lower abdominals, and hip flexors.

Purpose: Strengthen the core and hip flexor muscles. Improve balance and stability in the plank position.

What to Feel: Feel the engagement in your core as you lift each leg. Focus on maintaining a stable plank position. Emphasize the control of leg movements.

Advanced Wall Pilates Routines (15 minutes or less)

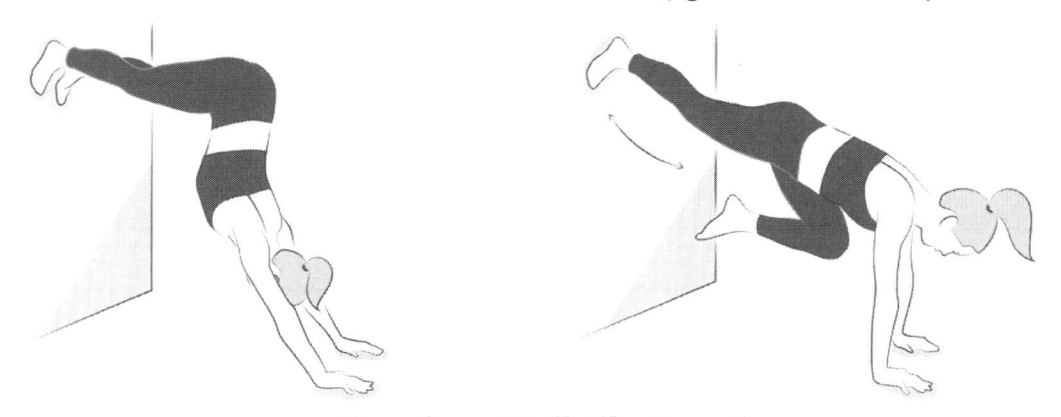

Exercise 1: Wall Pike Crunches

Get into a wall high plank, with both arms fully extended (with soft elbows) taking your weight and engage your core. Walk your hands to the left challenging your obliques and balance, then hold. Centre yourself and repeat on the other side.

Sets and Repetitions: 2 sets of 20 each side.

Targets: The core, especially transverse abdominus and obliques.

Purpose: Strengthen and tighten the entire core, including upper and lower abdominal muscles. Challenge the stability of the wall plank position.

What to Feel: Feel the contraction in your core as you hold positions. Focus on keeping your body braced in a straight line as you move. Emphasize a smooth and controlled movements from side to side.

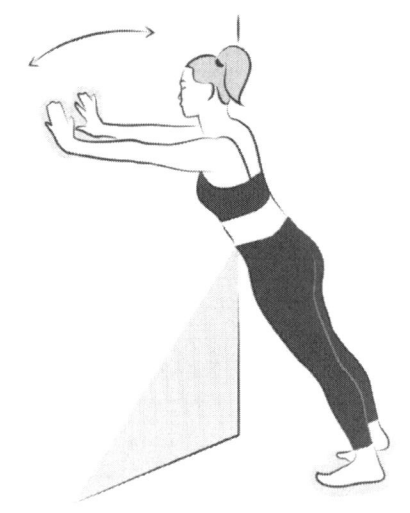

Exercise 2: Wall Plank with Arm Walk

Assume a wall plank position with hands on the floor. Lift your hips towards the ceiling, forming an inverted V shape. Bring your right knee towards your chest, then switch to the left. Continue for 40 seconds, then rest for 20 seconds.

Sets and Repetitions: 3 sets of lateral walks (10 seconds each side).

Targets: The core, shoulders, and stabilizing muscles.

Purpose: Enhance core strength and stability. Improve shoulder mobility. Challenge coordination and balance.

What to Feel: Feel the engagement in your core and shoulders during lateral walks. Focus on maintaining a straight body line. Emphasize control and precision in hand movements.

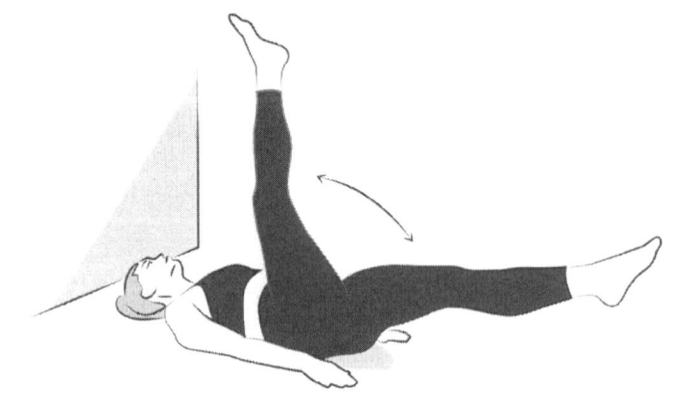

Exercise 3: Scissor Kicks

Lie on your back, hands pressed into the floor. Lift legs vertically and scissor them in controlled movements. Focus on pressing your lower back into the floor a little to further engage your core muscles.

Sets and Repetitions: Perform 2 sets of 20 scissor kicks.

Targets: The core and lower abdominal muscles.

Purpose: The purpose is to challenge the core with dynamic leg movements while lying on your back.

What to Feel: Focus on pressing your hands into the floor for stability and feel the engagement in your core as you scissor kick your legs vertically.

I'd like you to think of these 15-minutes or less workouts, as rounds in a circuit. If you only have a very short amount of time to exercise, focus on completing 1 or 2 quality rounds. If you have the full 15-minutes, try to fit in multiple rounds. As your body becomes fitter and stronger, you will be able to take less rest time between sets, and complete more rounds within the 15-minute time frame.

Concluding Musings: 15-Minute Wall Pilates Routines for Every Woman

In the hustle and bustle of modern life, prioritizing our health and fitness often takes a backseat to the myriad responsibilities we juggle daily. As discussed, these 15-minute Wall Pilates Routines offer a practical solution for those navigating tight schedules, providing an efficient and effective means to stay on track with fitness goals.

The significance of short and sharp workouts cannot be overstated, especially in a world where time is a precious commodity. These routines serve as quick and accessible tools, ensuring that even on the busiest days, we can carve out moments for self-care. Whether you are a beginner looking to establish a consistent practice, an intermediate enthusiast seeking variety, or an advanced practitioner aiming for a challenge, there's a tailored routine to fit every level.

The desire for slimmer, toned abs, more pronounced glutes, and lean arms and stomach is a shared aspiration among many women. The Wall Pilates Routines presented cater to these specific targets, acknowledging the common focus areas like triceps, tummy, and back fat. The routines not only address aesthetic goals but also contribute to overall well-being, promoting strength, flexibility, and core stability.

For beginners, the emphasis is on foundational movements and core activation, providing a solid starting point. Intermediate routines introduce more complexity, targeting multiple muscle groups and enhancing overall body strength. Advanced practitioners can challenge themselves with intricate exercises that demand increased coordination, balance, and endurance.

Incorporating these routines into our lives is a testament to prioritizing oneself amid the chaos. The flexibility of Wall Pilates, both in terms of time and location, makes it an ideal companion for women striving to achieve their fitness goals without compromising other commitments.

Let the 15-minute Wall Pilates Routines serve as a reminder that investing time in our well-being need not be an arduous task. With dedication and consistency, these routines become powerful tools in our journey towards achieving the coveted slimmer abs, toned booty, and lean body, aligning with the collective aspirations of many women. So, let us embrace the efficacy of short, targeted workouts and walk the path of a healthier, stronger, and more empowered version of ourselves.

As we conclude our exploration of the 15-minute Wall Pilates routine, the journey towards a healthier, more empowered you continues seamlessly into the next chapter, where we work through the Beginner Program which will span the first seven days of your fitness adventure.

FREE BONUS:
FULL VIDEO GUIDES

It can be tough leaning some exercises from a book. So with that in mind I have created video guides for each of the exercises featured in this chapter that you can access for free. Coupled with the teaching points within the book, you should find it super easy to correct your movements and get your form just right.

To access these, go to your internet browser and type in bit.ly/wall-pilates and I'll email them to you.

You can also scan the QR Code below with your cell phone camera and tap the little link that appears if you find that easier.

I give all the bonuses in this book for free to ensure that you can get the most out of every workout.

6

BEGINNER PROGRAM: DAY 1 - 7

Every journey begins with one thing: *Taking the first step.*

Reminiscing about the beginning of my own first 30-day Wall Pilates workout journey, the excitement and determination flood back as I reflect on the initial stages of the Beginner Program: Day 1 - 7. Each memory is a chapter in the story of my pursuit of slimmer, toned abs, a bigger booty, and leaner arms.

I remember how I was nervous.

Scared.

I didn't know if I could follow through with it.

Would Wall Pilates even work?

Yet, on that very first day, there was so much curiosity and commitment in the air. The wall, an unexpected but welcome companion, supported me through foundational exercises targeting my core, arms, and legs. The routines, though seemingly simple, proved perfect for a beginner like me, and the 15-minute duration eased me into the challenge.

The week unfolded with a series of exercises that brought both a burn and a sense of accomplishment. Wall Squats, Planks, Leg Lifts... every movement felt like a step closer to the physique I aimed for. The routines, thoughtfully structured for gradual progression, allowed me to build an amazing body shape, while boosting my self-confidence at the same time.

Looking back, I realize the incredible impact that short and sharp workouts make on your results. The program, with its strategic design, served as a reliable guide, keeping me on track even when time was tight. Those initial seven days laid a solid foundation, proving that consistent, focused efforts in areas like triceps, tummy, and battling back fat could yield significant results.

As I navigate the memories of Beginner Program: Day 1 - 7, I'm filled with anticipation for the chapters that lie ahead in my fitness journey. The journey has just begun, and with each passing day, I grow closer to the version of myself I aspire to be.

Discovering Strength: A Novice's Week in Wall Pilates

Taking on the Wall Pilates Beginner Program: Day 1 - 7 is an empowering step towards a healthier and stronger version of oneself. Here are some valuable tips to make the most out of the initial seven days:

- **Set Realistic Goals**: Begin with clear and achievable goals tailored to your fitness level. Whether it's focusing on core strength, toning arms, or enhancing overall flexibility, having specific objectives will keep you motivated throughout the program.
- **Prioritize Form Over Intensity**: Pay careful attention to your form during each exercise. It's more beneficial to perform movements with precision and control than to rush through them. Proper form ensures targeted muscle engagement and minimizes the risk of injury.

- **Listen to Your Body**: Everyone's body is unique, and what works for one person might not be suitable for another. Pay attention to how your body responds to the exercises. If something feels uncomfortable or painful, don't hesitate to modify the movement or seek guidance.
- **Consistency is Key**: The Beginner Program is designed to build a foundation for your fitness journey. Consistency is crucial, so aim to complete the daily routines without skipping any sessions. Regular practice will yield more noticeable results over time.
- **Stay Hydrated and Eat Well**: Fueling your body with the right nutrients is essential. Hydration and a balanced diet contribute significantly to your overall well-being and energy levels. Make sure to drink enough water and incorporate wholesome foods into your meals.
- **Celebrate Small Wins**: Acknowledge and celebrate even the smallest achievements. Whether it's holding a plank for a few extra seconds or feeling increased strength in your legs, recognizing these victories will keep you motivated and excited for the next challenge.
- **Incorporate Recovery Techniques**: Allow your body time to recover and prevent burnout. Incorporate gentle stretching, foam rolling, or even a short walk on rest days. Recovery is a crucial aspect of any fitness program, promoting muscle repair and overall resilience.
- **Connect with a Support System**: Share your fitness journey with friends, family, or fellow participants. Having a support system can provide encouragement, accountability, and shared experiences, making the journey more enjoyable.

Starting the Wall Pilates Beginner Program is a commitment to self-improvement. With these tips in mind, embrace each day as an opportunity to grow both physically and mentally stronger, laying the groundwork for a fulfilling and results driven fitness journey.

Beginner Program: Day 1 – 7

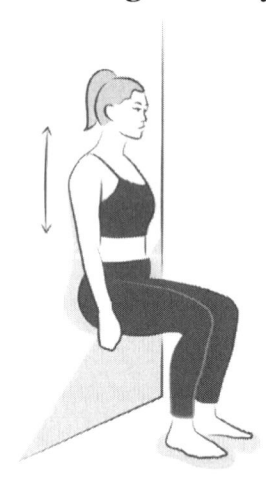

Exercise 1: Basic Core Activation

Stand with your back against the wall. Engage your core and slowly slide down the wall into a seated position. Hold the seated position for 30 seconds, focusing on maintaining core engagement. Slide back up the wall to the starting position.

Sets and Repetitions: 3 sets of 30 seconds sitting and 20 standing, alternating between seated and standing positions.

Targets: Core muscles, lower back, and legs.

Purpose: Activate and engage the core muscles, promoting stability and strength.

What to Feel: Focus on maintaining core engagement throughout the exercise.

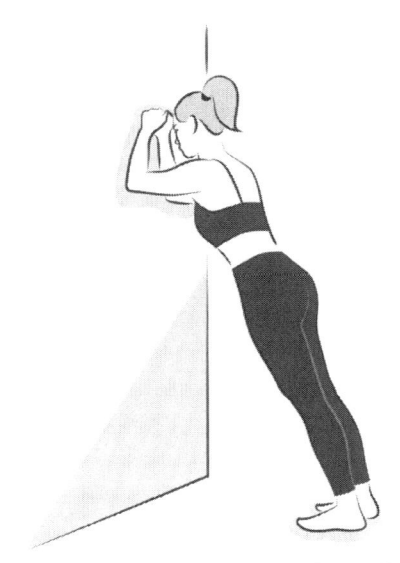

Exercise 2: Wall Plank Hold

Face the wall and place your hands on it, shoulder-width apart.

Step your feet back, creating a straight line from head to heels.

Hold the plank position for 40 seconds, engaging your core and glutes.

Rest for 20 seconds.

Sets and Repetitions: Hold the plank position for 40 seconds. Repeat 3 times.

Targets: Core muscles, shoulders, and glutes.

Purpose: Strengthen core and upper body, improve overall stability.

What to Feel: Engage the core and glutes, maintain a straight line from head to heels.

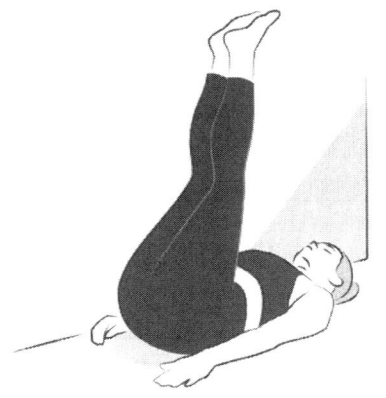

Exercise 3: Legs Up the Wall Stretch

Sit sideways next to the wall and swing your legs up, resting them against the wall.

Extend your arms to the sides for balance.

Hold the position for 30 seconds, feeling a gentle stretch in your hamstrings and lower back.

Lower your legs and rest for 10 seconds.

Sets and Repetitions: Hold the stretch for 30 seconds followed by 10 seconds of rest. Repeat once more.

Targets: Hamstrings and lower back.

Purpose: Stretch and release tension in the hamstrings and lower back.

What to Feel: Gentle stretch in hamstrings and lower back, focus on controlled.

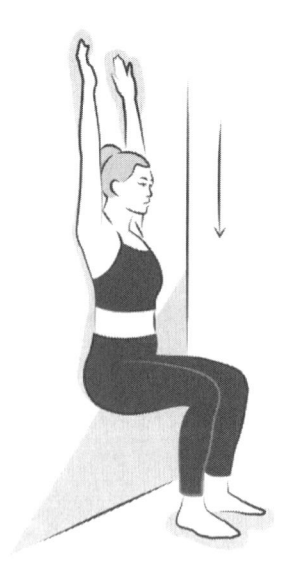

Exercise 4: Wall Squats with Arm Raises

Stand with your back against the wall. Lower into a squat position while simultaneously raising your arms overhead. Hold for 30 seconds, then return to the starting position. Rest for 15 seconds.

Sets and Repetitions: Hold the squat position for 30 seconds followed by 15 seconds of rest. Repeat for 3-4 repetitions.

Targets: Legs, glutes, shoulders, and arms.

Purpose: Engage lower body and shoulders, improve overall strength.

What to Feel: Engage core, feel the burn in legs, and arms.

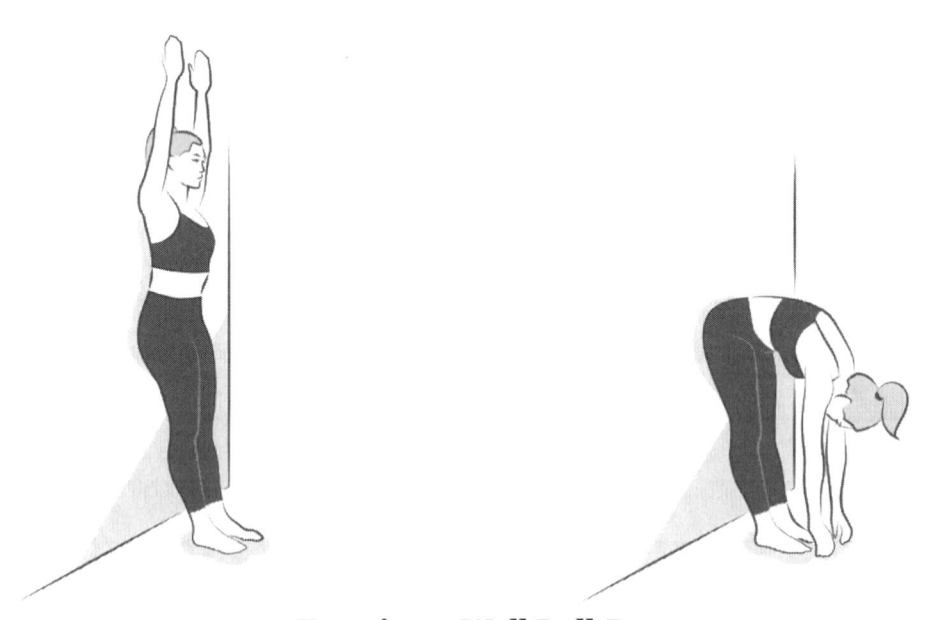

Exercise 5: Wall Roll-Downs

Stand against the wall with arms extended. Slowly roll the spine down, reaching towards the floor. Roll back up, engaging your core. Perform this movement for 40 seconds, then rest for 20 seconds.

Sets and Repetitions: Performing the roll-down for 40 seconds followed by 20 seconds of rest. Repeat for 2-3 repetitions.

Targets: Spine, core, and shoulders.

Purpose: Improve spine flexibility, engage core muscles.
What to Feel: Controlled articulation of the spine, engage core during the movement.

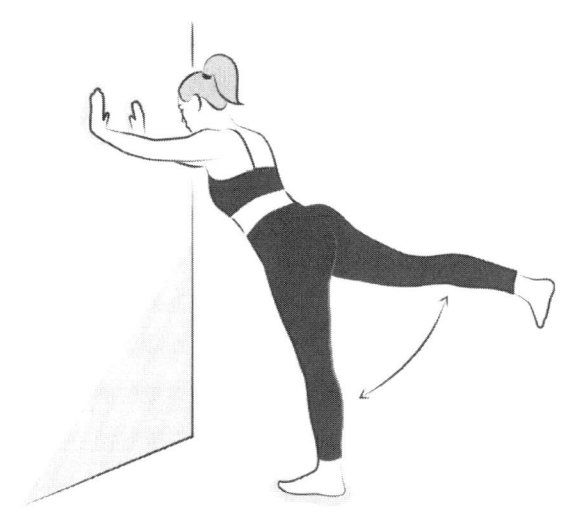

Exercise 6: Wall Plank with Leg Lifts

Start in a wall plank position. Lift one leg off the wall, keeping it straight. Hold for 20 seconds, then switch legs.
Sets and Repetitions: Repeat for 3-4 repetitions on each side, alternate legs. Repeat for 3-4 sets.
Targets: Core muscles, especially the lower abs.
Purpose: Strengthen core and lower abs, improve balance.
What to Feel: Engage core, feel the lift in the legs.

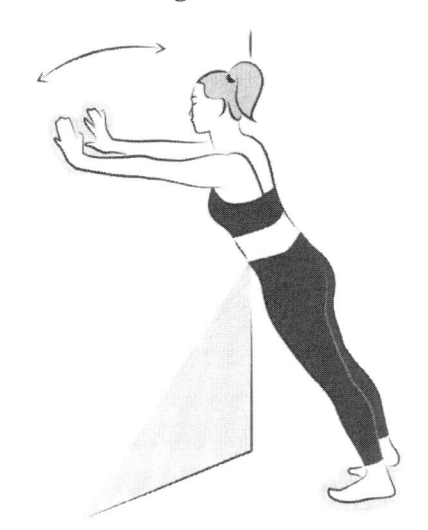

Exercise 7: Wall Plank with Arm Walk

Start in a wall plank position. Walk your hands laterally along the wall to the right for 10 seconds. Return to the center and repeat to the left.
Sets and Repetitions: Alternate arms for 4 reps each side. Repeat for 3-4 sets.
Targets: Core, shoulders, and arms.
Purpose: Improve core and upper body strength, enhance stability.
What to Feel: Engage core, feel the stretch in arms and shoulders.

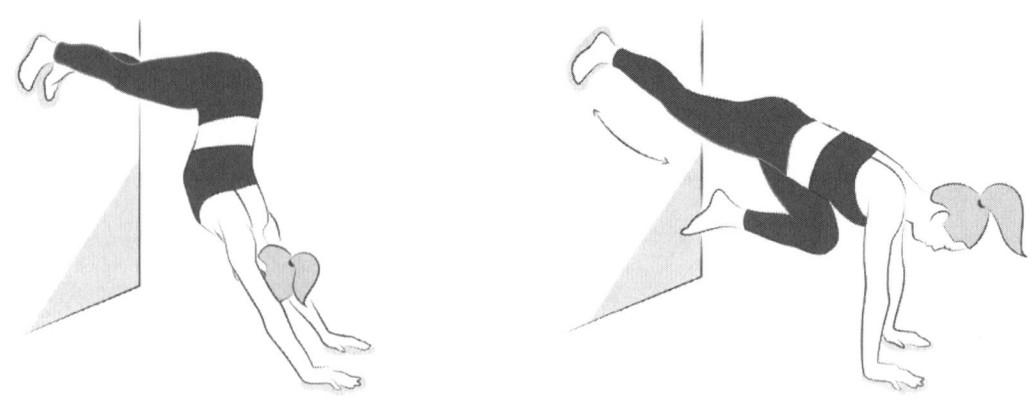

Exercise 8: Wall Pike Crunches

Assume a wall plank position with hands on the floor.

Lift your hips towards the ceiling, forming an inverted V shape. Bring your right knee towards your chest, then switch to the left. Continue for 40 seconds, then rest for 20 seconds.

Focus on controlled movements and engaging your core by drawing your abs in.

Sets and Repetitions: Continuous movement performing crunches for 40 seconds followed by 20 seconds of rest. Repeat for 3-4 sets.

Targets: Core muscles, especially upper abs.

Purpose: Strengthen core, particularly upper abs, and improve overall stability.

What to Feel: Engage core, feel the crunch in the upper abs.

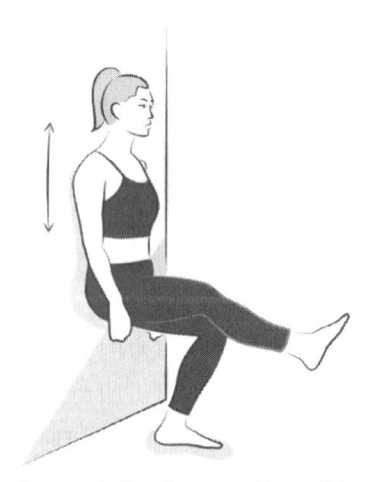

Exercise 9: Single-Leg Wall Squats

Stand on one leg with your back against the wall. Lower into a squat position, keeping one leg extended in front. Hold for 30 seconds, then switch legs.

Sets and Repetitions: Alternate legs, holding each squat position for 30 seconds with a 20 second rest between. Repeat for 3-4 sets.

Targets: Legs, glutes, and core.

Purpose: Engage lower body and core, improve balance.

What to Feel: Engage core, feel the burn in legs.

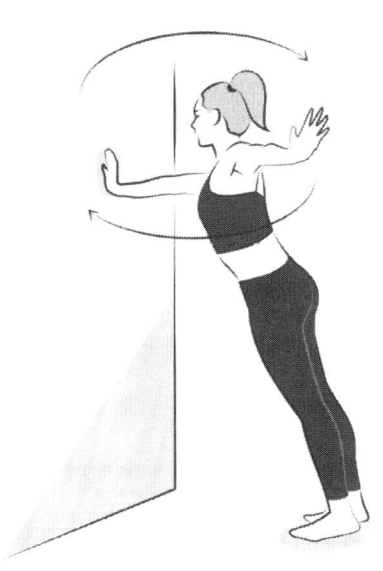

Exercise 10: Wall Plank with Arm Circles

Start in a wall plank position. Extend one arm forward and make small circles for 20 seconds.

Switch to the other arm and repeat. Focus on maintaining a stable plank position.

Sets and Repetitions: Make full circles for 20 seconds with one arm before switching to the opposite. Complete 2-4 repetitions on each side before resting for 20 seconds. Repeat for 2-3 sets.

Targets: Core, shoulders, and arms.

Purpose: Improve core and upper body strength, enhance stability.

What to Feel: Engage core, feel the circular motion in shoulders and arms.

Stepping Up: Transitioning to Intermediate Wall Pilates

Congratulations on successfully completing the Beginner Program: Day 1 - 7! You've laid a solid foundation for your Wall Pilates journey, embracing key exercises and focusing on building strength with precision. Now, it's time to elevate your practice to the next level.

Next up is the Intermediate Program: Day 8 - 14. This phase introduces a fresh set of exercises, offering new challenges and opportunities for growth. While the foundational principles remain, you'll notice a subtle shift in complexity, allowing you to further refine your technique and deepen your connection to the exercises.

The Intermediate Program marks a step up in your skill level and a leap forward in your results, and I'm excited for the progress and discoveries that lie ahead.

With that in mind, let's push forward together!

FREE BONUS:
EXERCISE CHARTS AND VIDEO GUIDES

To help you along on your Wall Pilates journey, I have put together fully illustrated exercise charts for your beginner program along with video guides to make sure that each movement you perform can be executed with precision to.

To access these, go to your internet browser and type in bit.ly/wall-pilates and I'll email them to you.

You can also scan the QR Code below with your cell phone camera and tap the little link that appears if you find that easier.

I give all the bonuses in this book for free to ensure that you can get the most out of every workout.

7

INTERMEDIATE PROGRAM: DAY 8 - 14

"You must become the change you want to see"

- MAHATMA GANDHI

"That was quite the workout, wasn't it?"

When I ask the question, the woman on the adjacent mat turns to smile at me.

Isabella, still catching her breath, nods in agreement. "Definitely challenging. I can feel the burn, for sure."

I nod, because she is right. I feel a pleasant burn in my muscles, evidence of a satisfying workout. The instructor's voice signals the end, and I take a moment to relish the sense of accomplishment.

I chuckle, "Same here. It's always tough, but so worth it in the end."

Isabella hesitates for a moment before admitting, "I don't know if I can keep this up. It's only been one week."

I place a reassuring hand on her shoulder, "Trust me, I felt the same way when I started. But here's the thing, that was just the beginner stage. It's time to up the difficulty and move on to the more challenging stage. You'll be amazed at how quickly your body adapts."

Encouraged, Isabella smiles and replies, "You think I can handle it?"

"Absolutely," I affirm. "You've got this. It's all about progress, not perfection. We'll tackle the next stage together."

As we gather our belongings, a shared determination replaces the initial exhaustion, and we leave the studio ready to face the increased challenge ahead.

Exploring Strength: Transitioning to Intermediate Wall Pilates

Venturing into the Intermediate Stage of Wall Pilates after completing the initial beginner program, marks a significant stride towards enhanced well-being and strength. When you feel ready to tackle the next phase of your program, here are essential insights to optimize your experience in the upcoming sessions:

- Gradual Progression: Understand that moving from beginner to intermediate is a gradual process. Don't rush it; let your body adapt and build strength over time.
- Listen to Your Body: Pay close attention to how your body responds to the increased intensity. If you experience pain (beyond normal muscle soreness), adjust the intensity accordingly and consult with an instructor.
- Consistent Attendance: Aim for regular attendance to maintain momentum. Consistency is key to progress in Pilates, especially as you advance to more challenging exercises.
- Hydrate and Fuel: Stay well-hydrated and ensure you're fueling your body with the right nutrients. Proper nutrition is crucial as the demands on your muscles increase.

- Engage Your Core: Focus on engaging your core muscles throughout each exercise. This becomes even more crucial in intermediate Pilates, as the movements become more intricate and challenging.
- Breathing Techniques: Pay attention to your breath. Coordinating your breath with each movement helps with control and enhances the effectiveness of the exercises.
- Utilize Props Mindfully: If props are introduced in intermediate Pilates, use them mindfully. They can add resistance and challenge but may also require additional coordination.
- Challenge Your Balance: Many intermediate exercises focus on balance. Embrace this challenge, as it not only strengthens your core but also improves overall stability.
- Ask Questions: Don't hesitate to ask an instructor for clarification or modification options. They're there to help you progress safely and effectively.
- Set Realistic Goals: Set achievable goals for yourself. Celebrate small victories along the way, while keeping in mind that progress may not always be linear.
- Stay Positive: Approach each session with a positive mindset. The mental aspect of Pilates is as important as the physical, and a positive attitude contributes to better performance.
- Rest and Recovery: Give your body the time it needs to recover. Adequate rest is essential for muscle growth and overall well-being.
- Self-Reflection: Take a moment after each session to reflect on what went well and where you can improve. This self-awareness will guide your ongoing progress.
- Enjoy the Journey: Pilates is a journey, not a destination. Enjoy the process of discovering what your body is capable of and savor the sense of accomplishment with each milestone.

Keep these guidelines in mind as you approach each session, welcoming every day as a chance to further develop your skill level and your body's ability to adapt and improve.

Intermediate Program: Day 8 – 14

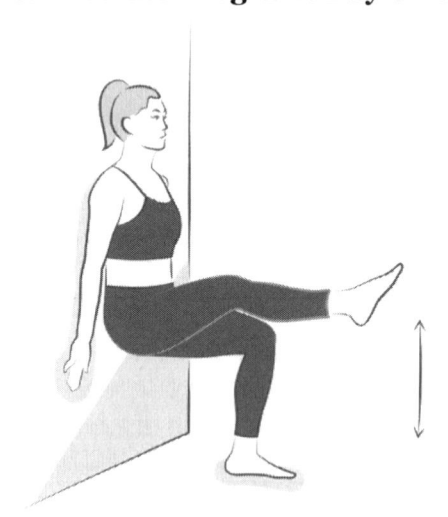

Exercise 1: Wall Sit Leg Lifts

Start with your back against the wall and legs in a seated position. Lift one leg at a time while maintaining the wall sit. Alternate between legs.

Sets and Repetitions: 3 sets of 12 reps per leg.

Targets: Focuses on quads, hamstrings, and core stability.

Purpose: Enhances lower body strength and stability.

What to Feel: Concentrate on engaging your core to maintain stability during leg lifts. Feel the burn in your thighs and challenge your balance.

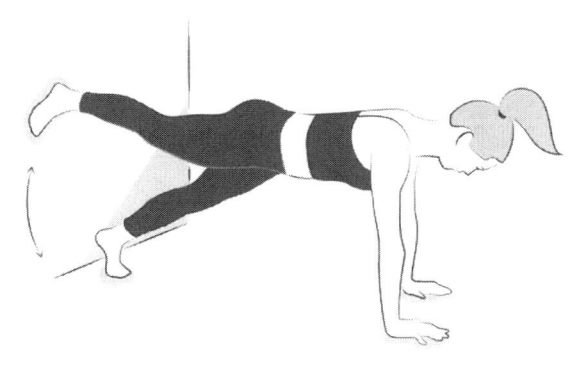

Exercise 2: Plank with Leg Extensions

Assume a plank position with your feet against the wall. Raise one leg higher to the wall at a time while keeping your body aligned.

Sets and Repetitions: 4 sets of 10 leg extensions per leg.

Targets: Engages core muscles, shoulders, and glutes.

Purpose: Strengthens the core and improves overall body control.

What to Feel: Focus on keeping your body in a straight line. Feel the contraction in your abs and the engagement in your glutes with each leg extension.

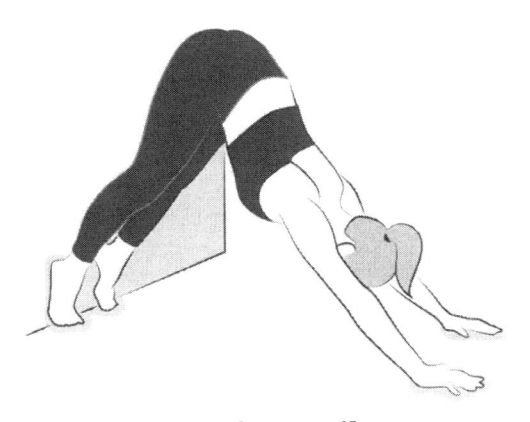

Exercise 3: Pike

Begin in a high plank position facing away from the wall. Slowly drive your hips upward toward the ceiling, forming an inverted V shape. Press your heels into the wall and keep your legs straight.

Sets and Repetitions: 4 sets of 12 reps.

Targets: Abdominals, shoulders, and hamstrings.

Purpose: Enhances core strength, shoulder stability, and hamstring flexibility.

What to Feel: Concentrate on the stretch in your hamstrings and the contraction in your core as you lift your hips.

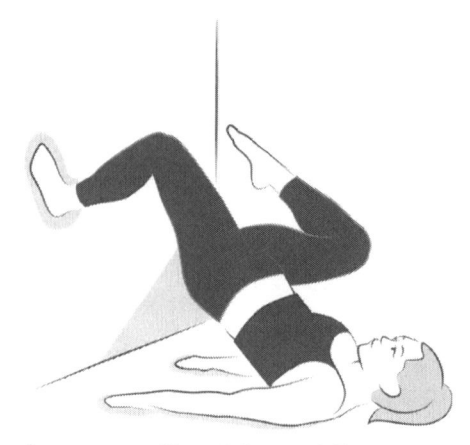

Exercise 4: Wall Bridge with Knee Tucks

Lie on your back with feet against the wall, lift your hips into a bridge position, then tuck your knees towards your chest.

Sets and Repetitions: 3 sets of 15 knee tucks.

Targets: Works on glutes, lower back, and abdominal muscles.

Purpose: Enhances core strength and glute activation.

What to Feel: Concentrate on squeezing your glutes at the top of the bridge. Feel the engagement in your lower abdominals during knee tucks.

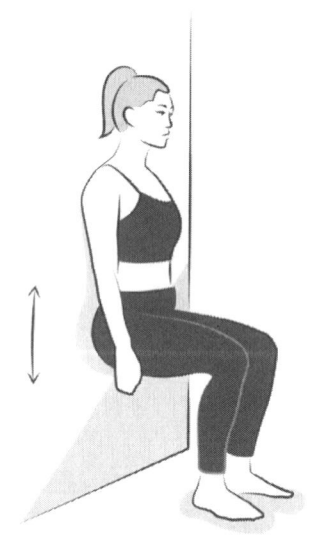

Exercise 5: Wall Squat Pulses

Stand against the wall, lower into a squat position, and pulse up and down within a small range.

Sets and Repetitions: 4 sets of 20 pulses.

Targets: Focuses on quads, hamstrings, and glutes.

Purpose: Builds lower body endurance and strength.

What to Feel: Keep the tension in your quads and glutes throughout the pulses. Feel the burn in your thighs.

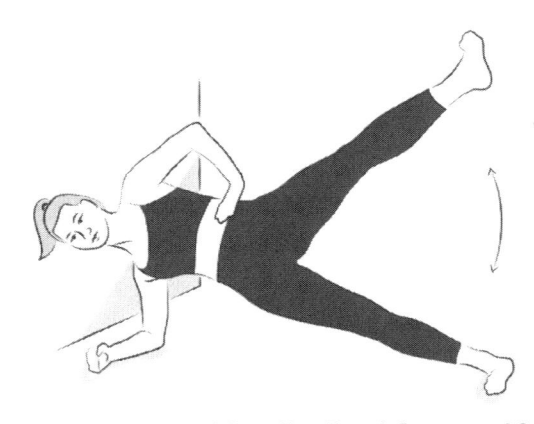

Exercise 6: Side Plank with Leg Lift

Form a side plank (with your elbow and forearm against the wall for support if needed). Lift the top leg up and down.

Sets and Repetitions: 3 sets of 12 leg lifts per side.

Targets: Engages obliques, hips, and outer thighs.

Purpose: Strengthens lateral core muscles and improves hip stability.

What to Feel: Focus on maintaining a straight line from head to toe. Feel the activation in your side muscles and outer thigh.

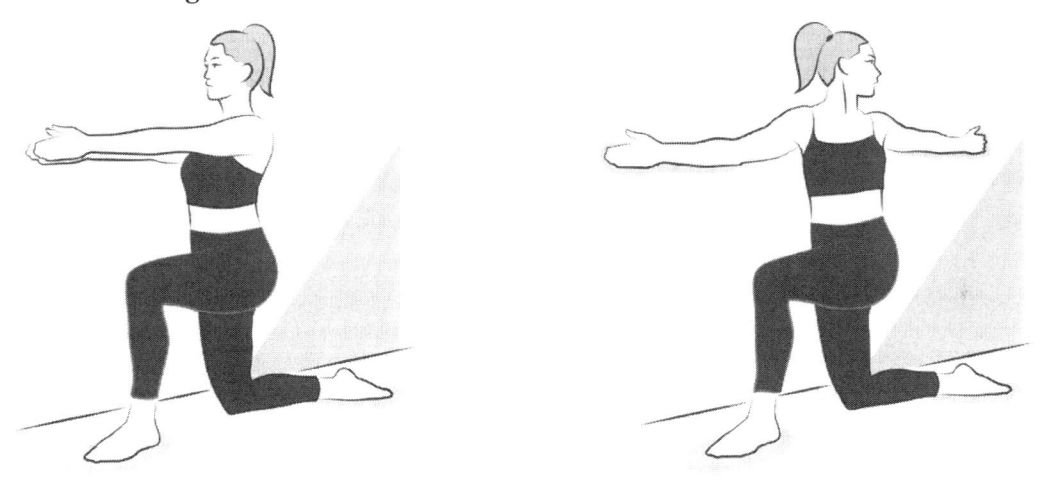

Exercise 7: Wall Rotation

In a lunge position with your knee closest to the wall on the floor and both arms extended in front (palms together).

Rotate your torso and separate your arms, expanding your chest, until both arms are touching the wall. Return to the start position under control.

Sets and Repetitions: Perform 2 sets of 15 rotations on each side.

Targets: The obliques and improves spinal mobility.

Purpose: The purpose is to strengthen the oblique muscles and enhance flexibility in the spine with controlled rotations against the wall.

What to Feel: Focus on keeping your back against the wall while rotating your torso from side to side. Feel the engagement in your obliques.

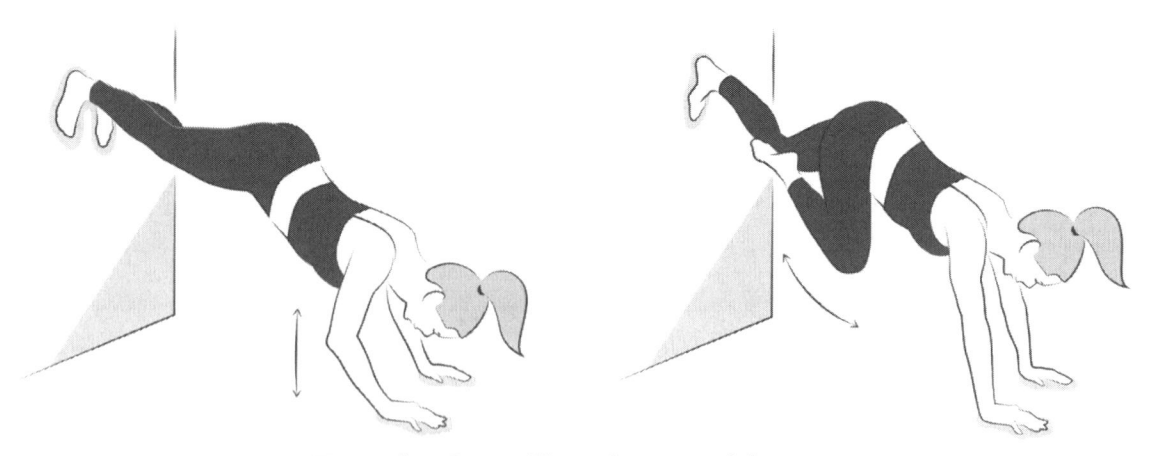

Exercise 8: Wall Push-Ups with Knee Tucks

Perform push-ups with hands against the wall. After each push-up, bring one knee towards your chest.

Sets and Repetitions: 3 sets of 15 push-ups with knee tucks.

Targets: Works on chest, triceps, and abdominal muscles.

Purpose: Strengthens upper body and core.

What to Feel: Maintain a straight line from head to toe during push-ups. Feel the contraction in your chest and abs during knee tucks.

Stepping Beyond: Transitioning to Advanced Mastery

As you triumphantly conquer the demanding exercises within the Intermediate Program, spanning from Day 8 to 14, you've undoubtedly marveled at the astonishing strides in both strength and endurance, not to mention the noticeable sculpting of that enviable booty!

Now, let's forge ahead with an Advanced Program. Brace yourself for this thrilling leap forward, where the exercises have been put together to further push your limits to new heights.

The Advanced Program is a bespoke adventure, artfully designed to unlock new dimensions of physical achievement and fortify your mental toughness. Prepare to further explore your capabilities as you push your body while learning the intricacies of advanced Wall Pilates exercises.

INTERMEDIATE PROGRAM: DAY 8 - 14

FREE BONUS:
EXERCISE CHARTS AND VIDEO GUIDES

Correct form is a major key to properly loading and ultimately shaping your body. To make sure that your form is always on point, I have included full video guides with accompanying exercise charts for your intermediate program for free.

To access these, go to your internet browser and type in bit.ly/wall-pilates and I'll email them to you.

You can also scan the QR Code below with your cell phone camera and tap the little link that appears if you find that easier.

I give all the bonuses in this book for free to ensure that you can get the most out of every workout.

8

ADVANCED PROGRAM: DAY 15 - 21

"You have to believe in yourself, challenge yourself, and push yourself until the very end; that's the only way you'll succeed"

- G-DRAGON

"Hey Eva! How was your wall Pilates class today?"

The juice bar's barista, Sophia, smiles at me. We've fallen into this routine. After an intense Wall Pilates session, I love to treat myself to a healthy smoothie to make the most of the workout.

I reply, still catching my breath, "Intense, but amazing! I'm in need of some post-workout nourishment. I'll go with the Green Bliss smoothie today, please."

Sarah nods, her hands deftly crafting the vibrant blend, which happens to be a concoction of kale, spinach, pineapple, and a touch of ginger for that extra kick.

"Excellent choice!" She says. "The Green Bliss is packed with antioxidants and nutrients. You're going to love it."

As I eagerly anticipate the refreshing blend, Sophia adds, "Anything else, Eva?"

I considered it for a moment and decided to add a sprinkle of chia seeds for that extra boost. "Yes, please, a sprinkle of chia seeds to top it off. Can't get enough of those omega-3s!"

With a final flourish, Sophia hands over the Green Bliss smoothie, and I take a blissful sip, relishing the cool, nutrient-packed goodness that perfectly complements the satisfying burn of a challenging wall Pilates workout.

As I sip on my smoothie, a familiar face, Lisa, approaches with a friendly smile. "Eva, we've been rocking those wall Pilates classes together for a while now. How does it feel, pushing ourselves through those workouts?"

I share a grin with her, appreciating the camaraderie we've developed in our fitness journey. "It's been an incredible journey, Lisa! The progress we've made is remarkable. I can feel my glutes getting toned and my abs getting tighter. The wall Pilates sessions have not only challenged us physically but also strengthened our bond as workout buddies."

Lisa nods in agreement, then leans in with a gleam of excitement in her eyes. "Do you think we're ready for the advanced level? I've been eyeing those challenging moves, and I think we can totally take them on together!"

Feeling a surge of enthusiasm, I reply, "Absolutely, Lisa! Let's embrace the challenge. We've conquered the intermediate phase, and I believe we're more than ready to elevate our game. Advanced wall Pilates, here we come!"

We share a high-five, energized by the prospect of pushing our limits and exploring new heights in our fitness journey.

Unleashing Power: Mastering Wall Pilates Challenges

Over the previous weeks you have focused on your form, on connecting your mind with your movements and developed your muscle tone, shape and flexibility. You are now at the stage where you are ready to tackle the Advanced Wall Pilates Program: Days 15 – 21. This marks another vital step forwards in your Wall Pilates regimen.

Here are some essential insights to help maximize the intensity and benefits of your advanced exercise sessions:

- Gradual Progression: Ease into the advanced wall Pilates exercises gradually. Start with a few advanced movements in each session and gradually increase the intensity as your strength and proficiency improve.
- Focus on Form: Pay meticulous attention to your form during advanced exercises. Precision is the key to reaping the full benefits and preventing injuries. Consider consulting with an instructor for guidance on proper technique.
- Increased Mind-Body Connection: Advanced wall Pilates requires an enhanced mind-body connection. Focus on every movement, engaging the targeted muscles consciously. This heightened awareness contributes to improved control and effectiveness.
- Challenge Your Limits: Embrace the challenge. Push yourself beyond your comfort zone by incorporating more challenging variations of familiar exercises. This can include adding props, increasing repetitions, or trying dynamic sequences.
- Consistency is Key: Consistency is crucial when transitioning to advanced levels. Aim for regular practice to build strength and proficiency. Set a schedule that aligns with your lifestyle, ensuring you dedicate time for advanced wall Pilates sessions.
- Incorporate Variety: Keep your routine dynamic by incorporating a variety of advanced exercises. This not only prevents monotony but also ensures that different muscle groups are engaged, contributing to overall strength and flexibility.
- Listen to Your Body: Advanced workouts can be demanding. Pay attention to your body's signals. If you experience discomfort beyond the normal burn, consider scaling back and gradually reintroducing challenging exercises as your body adapts.
- Professional Guidance: Seek guidance from a certified Pilates instructor or attend advanced classes to receive personalized feedback and corrections. Professional guidance ensures you perform the exercises correctly, maximizing effectiveness while minimizing the risk of injury.
- Set Clear Goals: Define specific goals for your advanced Wall Pilates journey. Whether it's mastering a challenging sequence or achieving specific strength milestones, clear goals provide motivation and a sense of accomplishment.
- Celebrate Achievements: Celebrate your progress and achievements along the way. Recognize the advancements in your strength, flexibility, and overall fitness. Positive reinforcement enhances motivation and keeps you committed to your advanced wall Pilates practice.

Advanced Program: Day 15-21

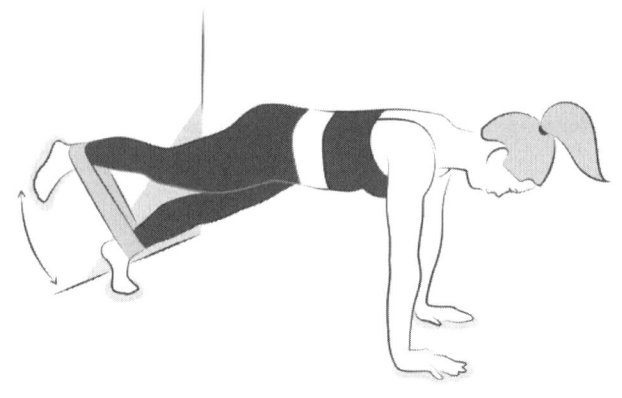

Exercise 1: Plank with Leg Extension and Resistance Band

Start in a plank position facing away from the wall, wrists directly under shoulders. Wearing a resistance band around your ankles, lift one leg off the floor, extending at the hips and keeping it straight.

Engage your core while maintaining a straight line from head to heel with your other leg. Alternate sides for each rep.

Sets and Repetitions: 3 sets of 10 reps on each leg.

Targets: Core muscles, glutes, and shoulders.

Purpose: Strengthens the core, improves balance, and tones the glutes.

What to Feel: Focus on maintaining stability in the plank position, feeling the engagement in your core and glutes.

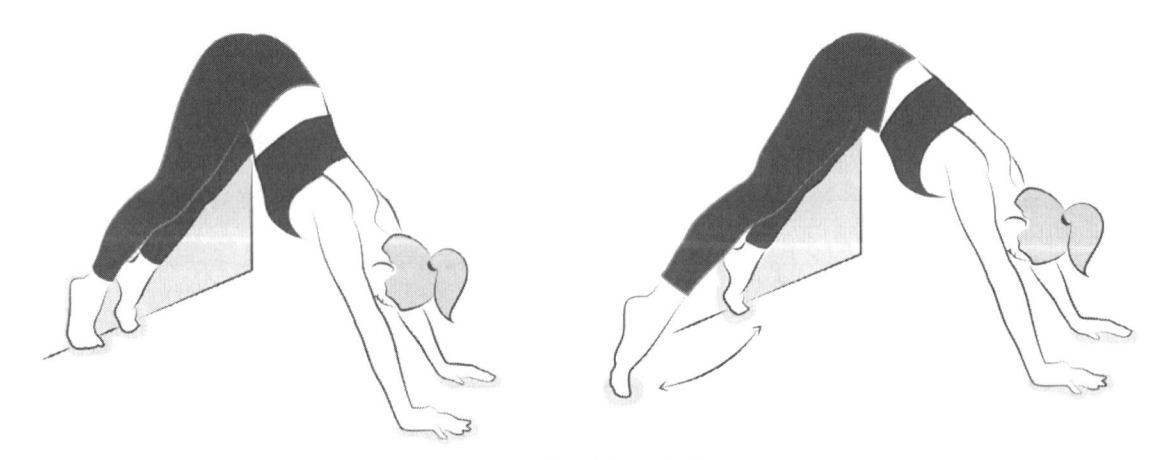

Exercise 2: Wall Pike with Leg Extension

Assume a plank position with feet against the wall. Lift your hips into a pike position. Extend left leg to the left, return. Then extend the right leg to the right and return. Repeat.

Sets and Repetitions: 4 sets of 10 leg extensions per leg.

Targets: Engages core muscles, shoulders, and hamstring flexibility.

Purpose: Strengthens the core and improves hamstring flexibility.

What to Feel: Focus on lifting your hips high into the pike. Feel the stretch in your hamstrings during leg extensions.

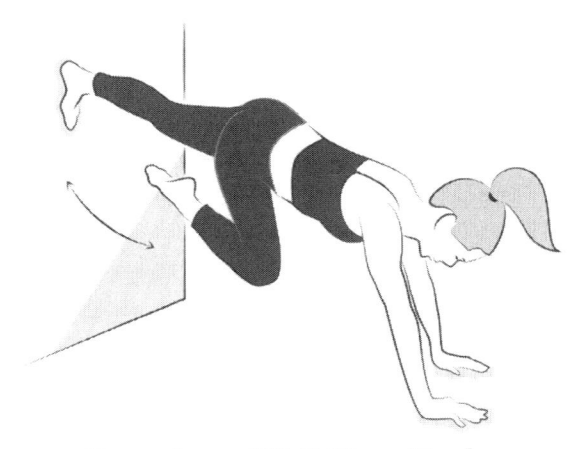

Exercise 3: Wall Knee Tucks

Start in a plank position facing the wall. Draw one knee towards your chest, rounding your spine. Extend the leg back to the starting position.

Sets and Repetitions: 3 sets of 15 reps on each leg.

Targets: Abdominals, hip flexors, and lower back.

Purpose: Improves abdominal strength and hip mobility.

What to Feel: Focus on the crunching motion in your abdominals as you bring your knee toward your chest.

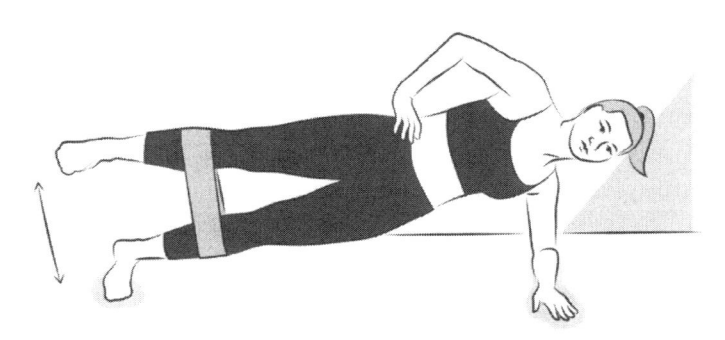

Exercise 4: Side Plank with Leg Lift and Resistance Band

Begin in a side plank position, supporting your weight on one forearm. With the resistance band around the ankles, lift the top leg toward the ceiling while keeping your core engaged.

Sets and Repetitions: 3 sets of 12 reps on each side.

Targets: Obliques, hips, and outer thighs.

Purpose: Strengthens the side muscles, improves hip stability, and tones the outer thighs.

What to Feel: Concentrate on the lift in your hips and the engagement in your obliques.

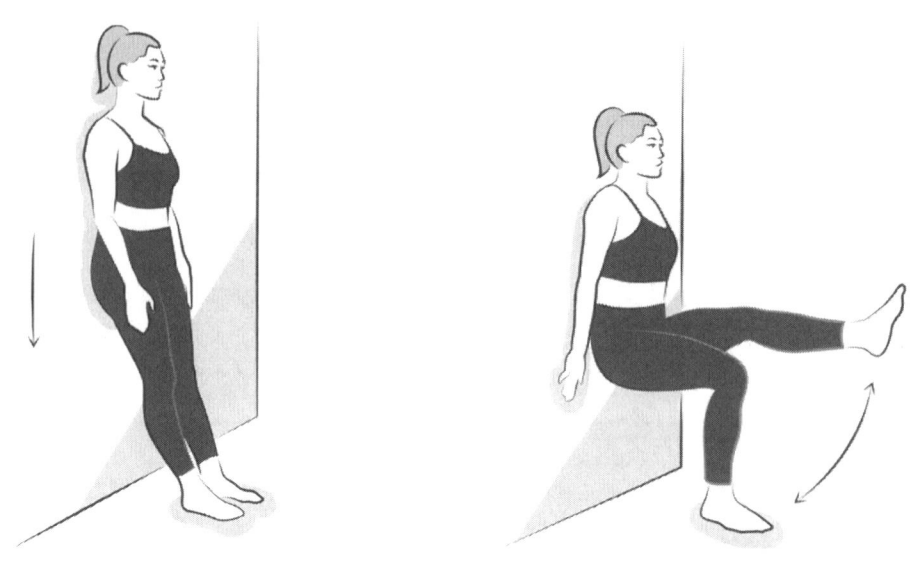

Exercise 5: Single-Leg Wall Sit

Stand with your back against the wall and lower into a squat position. Lift one leg, holding it parallel to the ground while maintaining the wall sit position.

Sets and Repetitions: 4 sets of 20 seconds on each leg.

Targets: Quadriceps, hamstrings, and glutes.

Purpose: Builds lower body strength and stability.

What to Feel: Focus on the burn in your quadriceps and the challenge of maintaining the wall sit with one leg lifted.

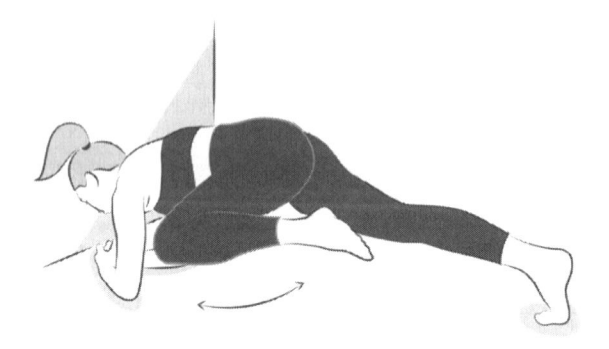

Exercise 6: Spiderman Plank

Start in a plank position facing the wall. Bring one knee towards the outside of the same elbow to engage your obliques. Return to a plank position and repeat on the other side.

Sets and Repetitions: 4 sets of 10 reps on each side.

Targets: Abdominals, obliques, and hip flexors.

Purpose: Works on core strength, oblique activation, and hip mobility.

What to Feel: Focus on the rotation and crunching motion as you bring your knee towards your elbow.

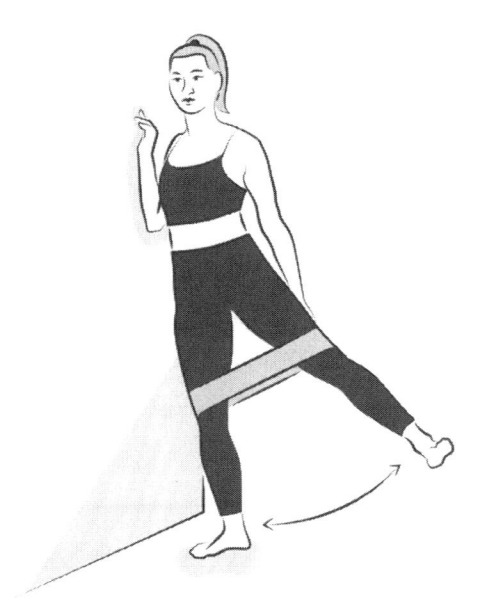

Exercise 7: Wall Lateral Leg Raises with Resistance Band

Stand sideways to the wall, placing one hand on it for support. Lift the top leg laterally, keeping it straight. Lower it back down with control.

Sets and Repetitions: 3 sets of 15 reps on each leg.

Targets: Abductors, outer thighs, and hip stabilizers.

Purpose: Tones the outer thigh muscles and improves hip stability.

What to Feel: Concentrate on the lift in your outer thigh and the engagement in your hip stabilizers.

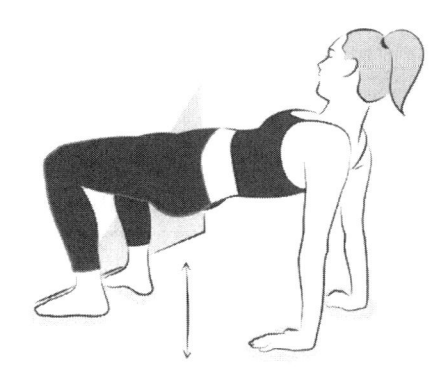

Exercise 8: Reverse Plank

Sit with your feet against the wall and hands placed on the floor. Lift your hips towards the ceiling, forming a reverse plank position that looks like a "table". Keep the toes pointing forward and squeeze the glutes at the peak of each movement.

Sets and Repetitions: 4 sets of 15 seconds hold.

Targets: Core muscles, shoulders, and glutes while extending the hip flexors.

Purpose: Strengthens the posterior chain, improves shoulder stability, and engages the core.

What to Feel: Concentrate on the lift in your hips and the activation in your core and shoulders.

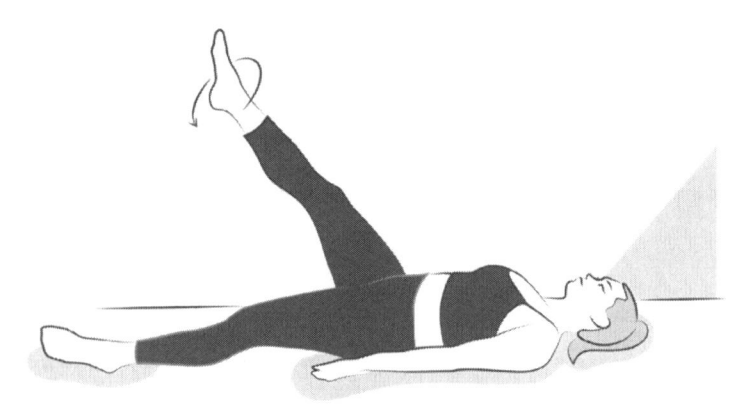

Exercise 9: Leg Circle

Lie on your back with your legs extended. Raise one leg and while keeping it straight, make small circles it in a clockwise motion, and then do the reverse before switching to the opposite leg.

Sets and Repetitions: 3 sets of 10 circles in each direction for each leg.

Targets: Abdominals, hip flexors, and inner thighs.

Purpose: Enhances core stability, hip mobility, and inner thigh strength.

What to Feel: Focus on the controlled circular movement of each leg, engaging your core and inner thighs.

Pushing Boundaries: Navigating Complexity by Finishing Strong

As you push through the demanding exercises within the Advanced Program, reflect on the remarkable strides achieved in strength and endurance that you've made. Revel in the transformation, not just in your overall physical shape but in particular the sculpting of your abs and booty!

Prepare to be exhilarated by your next leap forward, where the exercises and programs have been meticulously crafted to magnify both intensity and complexity, purposefully pushing your limits to unprecedented heights. The next set of Advanced Program exercises promises to unlock new dimensions of physical achievement while strengthening your mental toughness.

Your unwavering dedication has laid a robust foundation for this next chapter. Together, let's ascend to new heights, taking your fitness journey up another notch in the upcoming days. Embrace the challenge and know that each hurdle will bring you newfound strength, further enhance your shape and sense of grace. I'm sure that as your Wall Pilates journey continues, you can see that the possibilities for improving your body are limitless.

FREE BONUS:
VIDEO GUIDES AND EXERCISE CHARTS

As we have discussed throughout this book, to get maximum effectiveness out of every one of your workouts, you must make sure that you move through your full range under total controlled. This will load your muscles correctly leading to long, lean and sculpted muscles. To help you maintain your form and keep everyone of your movements awesome, I have included full video guides with exercise charts for free to accompany this chapter.

To access these, go to your internet browser and type in bit.ly/wall-pilates and I'll email them to you.

You can also scan the QR Code below with your cell phone camera and tap the little link that appears if you find that easier.

I give all the bonuses in this book for free to ensure that you can get the most out of every workout.

9

FINISH STRONG! DAY 22 - 28

"Life isn't about finding yourself. Life is about creating yourself."

- GEORGE BERNARD SHAW

"Eva, can you believe how far we've come?" Heather remarks, her eyes reflecting a mix of amazement and pride.

As I stand outside the Wall Pilates studio, the cool breeze carries a sense of accomplishment. I turn to Heather, who is equally as excited.

I chuckle, "Right? I never thought Pilates could do so much. My booty's perkier, abs are sculpted, and I feel a whole new level of strength."

Heather nods in agreement, "It's not just physical, though. I've noticed a boost in confidence too. It's incredible how these exercises work wonders for both body and mind."

Sharing our stories, we celebrate the newfound resilience and vitality we've gained through Wall Pilates. It's more than a fitness routine; it's a journey that has brought positive transformations, and the sense of accomplishment resonates in every word we exchange.

As we bask in the glow of our achievements, Heather and I share a glance filled with determination. "You know," Heather suggests with a spark in her eyes, "I think we're ready for the next level. Something more challenging, pushing our limits even further."

I nod in agreement, feeling the excitement building.

"Absolutely! Let's add some weights and take it up a notch. I'm all in for finishing strong," I respond, a newfound enthusiasm evident in my voice.

With a shared resolve, we decide to embrace the challenge, welcoming the idea of incorporating weights into our Wall Pilates routine. The prospect of pushing ourselves to new heights and finishing strong ignites a sense of anticipation for the exhilarating journey ahead.

Beyond Boundaries: The Grand Finale of Wall Pilates Mastery

As we stand on the brink of the final leg of our Wall Pilates challenge, the reflection on our journey so far brings a sense of accomplishment. From the tentative steps of the beginners to the intricate moves of the advanced phase, the transformation is undeniable. The wall has witnessed our dedication, shaping not only our bodies but also our resilience and commitment.

Now, with a steely resolve, we decide it's time to step it up a notch. We've conquered the fundamentals, navigated the complexities, and sculpted a stronger version of ourselves. It's only fitting that we introduce additional equipment and weights into our regimen, elevating the challenge and pushing our boundaries even further.

As the walls echo with the determination in our hearts, we embrace the prospect of this final chapter. The clink of weights and the hum of new equipment become our anthem, signaling the beginning of a phase that promises to test our limits and crown our efforts with unparalleled strength and endurance.

This is not just the last leg; it's the grand finale, and we're ready to conquer it all.

Are Weights Right for You?

An excellent way to increase the challenge when practicing Wall Pilates is to add weights and other complicated equipment. But, you might not have weights, or don't want to use weights.

While adding weights can indeed amplify the challenge, there are alternative approaches for individuals without access to weights or those who prefer a weight-free workout. Incorporating variations in body positioning, adjusting angles, and focusing on controlled, deliberate movements can effectively elevate the difficulty level.

Ultimately, the key lies in continuously challenging your body with progressive movements and maintaining precision in your Pilates practice. Whether incorporating weights or relying on another method, the goal is to tailor the workout to your fitness level, preferences, and available resources.

Pros of Using Weights	**Possible Cons of Using Weights**
Increased Intensity: Adding weights to your Wall Pilates routine can elevate the overall intensity of the workout, leading to greater strength and endurance gains. **Muscle Engagement**: Weights engage different muscle groups, allowing for a more comprehensive full-body workout. **Versatility**: Dumbbells or resistance bands can add versatility to your exercises, enabling a wide range of movements and targeting specific muscle areas. **Progressive Challenge**: Incorporating weights provides an opportunity for progressive overload, helping you continuously challenge and improve your fitness level.	**Risk of Injury**: Incorrect use of weights or choosing ones that are too heavy may increase the risk of injury, especially if proper form is not maintained. **Strain on Joints**: Weights can put additional strain on joints, and individuals with joint issues or injuries should be cautious when incorporating them. **Decreased Range of Motion**: In some exercises, weights might limit the range of motion, hindering the effectiveness of certain Pilates movements. **Complexity**: Introducing weights can add complexity to the workout, which you might not want if you value simplicity.

Deciding Whether Weights are Right for You

Physical Condition: Individuals with existing joint or health issues should consult with a fitness professional or healthcare provider before adding weights.

Fitness Goals: If your goal is to enhance muscle strength and endurance, weights could be beneficial. However, if you prioritize flexibility and bodyweight control, they may not be necessary.

Note: Always prioritize proper form and safety when introducing weights into your Wall Pilates routine. Consulting with a fitness professional can help tailor the use of weights to your specific needs and goals.

No Weights? No Problem

Use this list as a guide if you do not have weights, or choose not to use them.

Bodyweight Resistance:
- **How to**: Focus on controlled movements using your body weight for resistance. Engage core muscles to intensify exercises.
- **Targets**: Full-body engagement, core strength, and endurance.
- **Purpose**: Building strength and stability without the need for external weights.
- **What to feel**: Emphasize muscle engagement and maintain proper form throughout the movements.

Increased Repetitions:
- **How to**: Perform more repetitions of each exercise to create fatigue and challenge muscles.
- **Targets**: Muscular endurance and toning.
- **Purpose**: Elevating the intensity without adding external resistance.
- **What to feel**: Gradual fatigue and a deepening burn in targeted muscle groups.

Extended Hold Times:
- **How to**: Increase the duration of static holds during exercises like planks or leg lifts.
- **Targets**: Isometric strength and endurance.
- **Purpose**: Enhancing the challenge by sustaining muscle contraction over an extended period.
- **What to feel**: Focus on maintaining proper form and feeling the muscles working throughout the hold.

Varied Range of Motion:
- **How to**: Modify the range of motion during exercises, such as deepening squats or lunges.
- **Targets**: Muscular flexibility and strength through a full range of motion.
- **Purpose**: Increasing difficulty without additional weights.
- **What to feel**: Controlled movements with emphasis on muscle engagement.

Dynamic Movements:
- **How to**: Incorporate dynamic and complex Pilates movements like scissor kicks, teasers, or advanced variations.
- **Targets**: Balance, coordination, and overall body control.
- **Purpose**: Introducing complexity to challenge the body without external resistance.
- **What to feel**: Increased demand on core stability and coordination.

Increased Exercise Complexity:
- **How to**: Progress to more intricate variations of traditional Pilates exercises.
- **Targets**: Core strength, balance, and coordination.
- **Purpose**: Advancing the difficulty level through complex movements.
- **What to feel**: Heightened concentration and engagement in the targeted muscles.

Resistance Bands:
- **How to**: Incorporate resistance bands for added challenge without using traditional weights.
- **Targets**: Muscle groups specific to the chosen exercises.
- **Purpose**: Adding external resistance without the need for dumbbells or kettlebells.

What to feel: Increased resistance during movements.

Finish Strong Program: Day 22 – 28

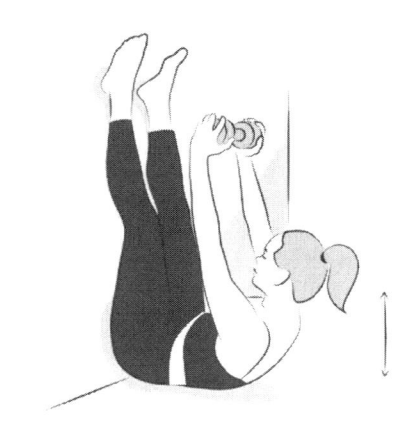

Exercise 1: Weighted Wall Teaser

Lie on your back, legs against the wall, holding a weight. Lift arms and weight upward, reaching for toes. Lower back down with control.

Sets and Repetitions: 4 sets of 10 reps.

Targets: Abdominals, hip flexors, and overall core.

Purpose: Develop core strength and control with the added challenge of holding a weight.

What to Feel: Deep contraction in the abs, a stretch through the hip flexors, and the resistance of the weight.

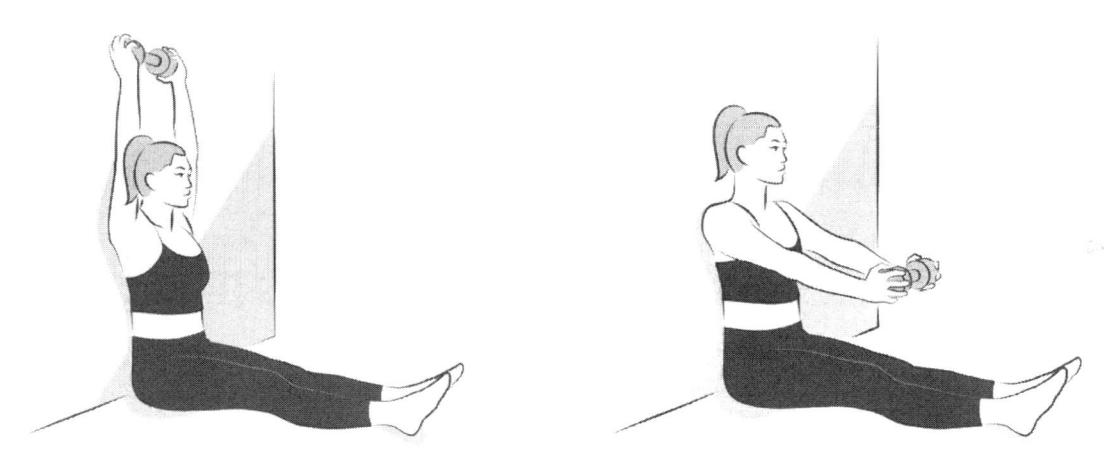

Exercise 2: Weighted Wall L-Sit

Sit on the floor, back against the wall, with legs extended, holding a weight. Move your arms and weight toward your toes. When you reach your arms back up, hold the L-shaped position.

Sets and Repetitions: 4 sets, hold for 20 seconds each.

Targets: Core, quadriceps, and hip flexors.

Purpose: Build isometric strength in the core and lower body while managing weight.

What to Feel: Intense contraction in the abdominal area, engagement in thighs, and the challenge of the added weight.

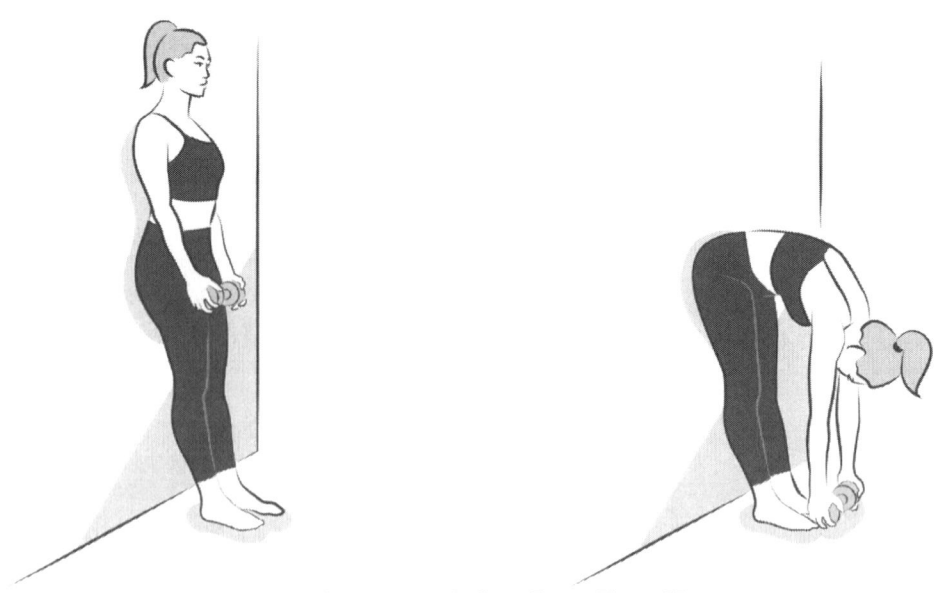

Exercise 3: Weighted Wall Roll-Down

Start standing up, back and legs against the wall, holding a weight. Roll down, reaching for toes. Roll back up with control.

Sets and Repetitions: 3 sets of 12 reps.

Targets: Abdominals, spinal flexors, and hip flexors.

Purpose: Enhance core flexibility and control during the movement while managing the additional weight.

What to Feel: Sequential activation of abdominal muscles throughout the roll-up, with the resistance of the weight.

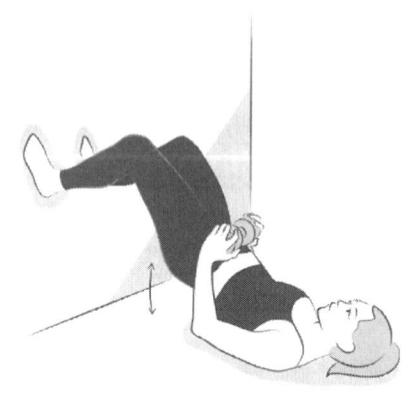

Exercise 4: Weighted Wall Glute Bridge

Lie on your back, legs up against the wall, holding a weight. Thrust your hips off the ground, bringing your legs overhead. Lower back down with control.

Sets and Repetitions: 3 sets of 10 reps.

Targets: Lower abs, hip flexors, and spinal extensors.

Purpose: Develop strength in the lower abdominal region and improve spinal mobility with added resistance.

What to Feel: Intense activation in the lower abs, a stretch in the spine, and the challenge of the weight.

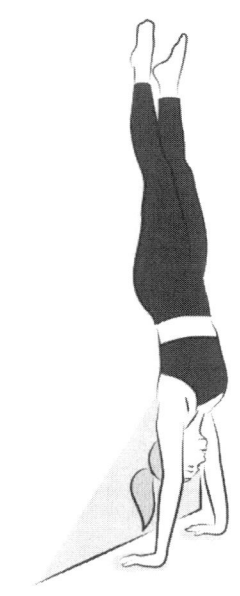

Exercise 5: Wall Handstand Hold

Kick up into a handstand position with your back against the wall. Hold the handstand position.

Sets and Repetitions: 3-5 sets, hold for up to 30 seconds.

Targets: Shoulders, core, and overall body stability.

Purpose: Enhance shoulder strength and balance with the added challenge of weights.

What to Feel: Activation in the shoulders and a sense of balance, managing the weight.

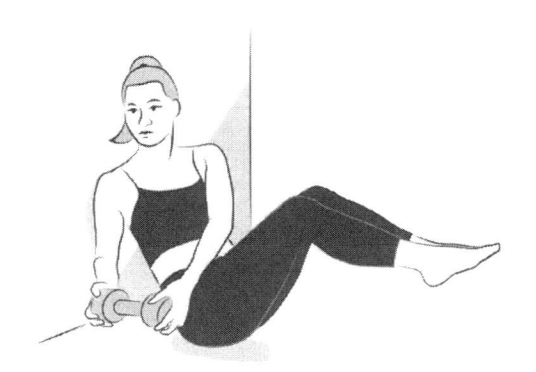

Exercise 6: Weighted Oblique Twist

Sit on the floor, holding a weight in both hands. Lean back slightly, touching the wall with your upper back for support if needed. Twist the torso smoothly to one side, then the other passing the weight over your lap.

Sets and Repetitions: 4 sets of 20 twists (10 each side).

Targets: Obliques and lateral core muscles.

Purpose: Improve rotational strength and flexibility with added resistance.

What to Feel: Contraction in the obliques with each twist and the challenge of the weight.

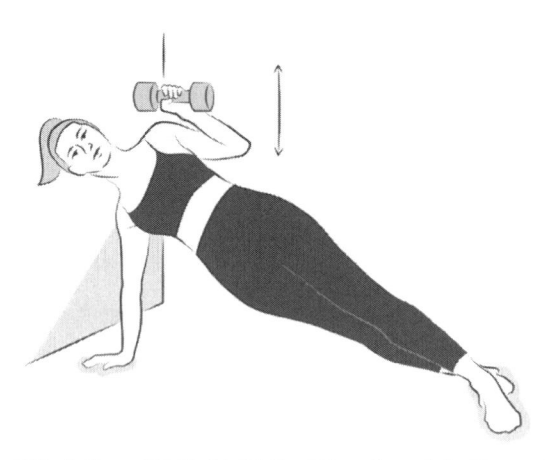

Exercise 7: Weighted Wall Side Plank with Dumbbell Raise

Assume a side plank position with feet against the wall, holding a dumbbell in the top hand. Lift the dumbbell towards the ceiling, maintaining balance. Lower the dumbbell with control.

Sets and Repetitions: 3 sets of 15 reps on each side.

Targets: Shoulders, obliques, and lateral core.

Purpose: Improve shoulder stability and oblique strength with the added challenge of a weight.

What to Feel: Activation in the shoulders, side body engagement, and the resistance of the weight.

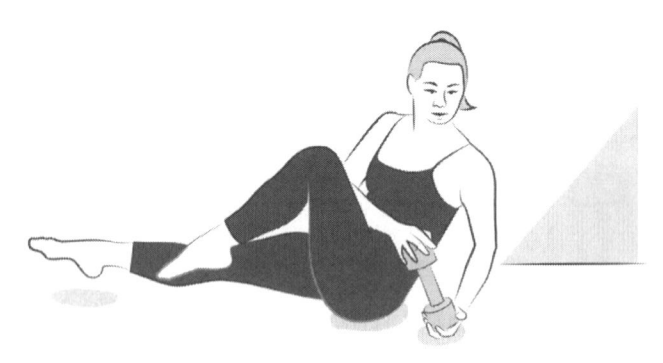

Exercise 8: Weighted Wall Bicycle Crunches

Lie on your back, legs against the wall, holding a weight. Perform bicycle crunches by bringing one knee towards the chest while twisting the torso. Alternate sides.

Sets and Repetitions: 3 sets of 20 reps (10 each side).

Targets: Abdominals, obliques, and hip flexors.

Purpose: Intensify traditional bicycle crunches by incorporating a weight for added resistance.

What to Feel: Activation in the abs and obliques during each twist, engagement in hip flexors, and the challenge of the weight.

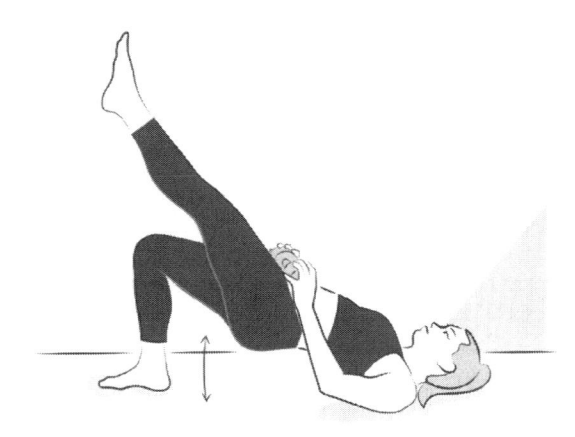

Exercise 9: Weighted Single Leg Glute Bridge

Lie on your back, holding a weight over your hips. Lift one leg towards the ceiling and then thrust hips upward focusing on keeping your hips level. Complete 10 reps. Repeat with other leg.

Sets and Repetitions: 4 sets of 10 reps on each side.

Targets: Lower abs, hip flexors, and glutes.

Purpose: Develop lower abdominal strength, hip flexor flexibility, and glute activation with the challenge of added weight.

What to Feel: Contraction in the lower abs, engagement in the glutes, and the challenge of the weight.

FREE BONUS:
VIDEO GUIDES AND EXERCISE CHARTS

Now that was a tough workout! Just like in the previous chapters, I have included full video guides with exercise charts for free to accompany this chapter.

To access these, go to your internet browser and type in bit.ly/wall-pilates and I'll email them to you.

You can also scan the QR Code below with your cell phone camera and tap the little link that appears if you find that easier.

I give all the bonuses in this book for free to ensure that you can get the most out of every workout.

10

HUSTLE AND TONE
SHORT WORKOUTS FOR A BUSY LIFE

"Good things happen to those who hustle."

— ANAIS NIN

As I stroll down the busy city street, months after completing my 28-day Wall Pilates challenge, I spot Heather in the distance.

Wow, I think, *so much has changed.*

She's pushing a baby carriage, juggling groceries, and looks visibly overwhelmed. Making my way toward her, memories of our fitness journey flood my mind, and I can't help but smile at the memories of how we ended our Pilates challenge.

"Heather!" I call out, catching her attention. "Long time no see! How's everything going?"

She glances up, a mixture of exhaustion and relief crossing her face. "Eva! Oh, it's been a whirlwind. This little one keeps me on my toes, and these groceries aren't making it any easier."

We exchange a quick hug, and I offer to lend a hand with the groceries. As we walk together, Heather opens up about the challenges of motherhood and finding time for herself amid the chaos. I can't help but reflect on the mental and physical strength we cultivated during our Pilates journey.

"You know, Heather, Pilates isn't just about the 28 days. It's about building lasting strength and resilience. How have you been keeping up with Wall Pilates?"

Heather sighs, a hint of disappointment in her voice. "Honestly, Eva, I fell off the Wall Pilates routine. Life got so hectic with the baby, work, and everything else. I just couldn't keep up with it all."

I nod understandingly, recognizing the challenges many face in maintaining a fitness routine amidst a busy life. "It's completely understandable, Heather. Life can throw curveballs, especially with a little one around."

She nods. "Tell me about it."

"I totally get how busy life can get, especially with a little one," I sympathize. "But it doesn't mean that we give up. Guess what? I've got your back."

Her eyes light up. "What do you have in mind?"

"I've prepared some quick and effective workouts that you can easily squeeze into your schedule. How about giving these a try?"

"Okay," Heather asks. "What are they?"

"Well, first there's the 10-Minute Ab Sculpting Core Blast."

"Sounds intense."

"It is!" I say. "It's a fast-paced and intense workout that targets and strengthens your abs. Yeah, it'll make you feel the burn, but trust me when I say that the results are totally worth it!"

Heather smiles. "It would definitely help me get back into things. What else do you have?"

"There's the 15-Minute Glute Focused Booty Builder: Time to bring back that sculpted booty! This workout specifically hones in on your glutes, giving you that extra boost of confidence."

Heather says, "Love it! What about toning my legs?"

"Well," I say, "There's the 10-Minute Legs and Arms Toning Workout... An efficient combo to tone both your legs and arms. Perfect for working on multiple areas in a short amount of time."

Heather already seems more relaxed and confident. "I love this!" she exclaims.

"Great!" I encourage. "Just remember, these workouts are designed to be quick yet super effective. Take them at your own pace, and know that I'm here to support you every step of the way. Best of luck, and let's reignite that Wall Pilates glow together!"

...

When beginning any fitness journey and while highly motivated, many women, like Heather, start a Pilates routine or challenge with fervor, only to find themselves slipping back into old habits due to life's demands. The struggle to stay consistent is real, and I understand it. That's why this chapter is here to provide you with valuable tricks and tips to maintain your commitment to Wall Pilates, even on the busiest days.

Consistency is key, and I'll share insights on how to seamlessly integrate Pilates into your daily routine. Life is hectic, and we all face time constraints, but fear not! I've curated quick and effective workouts tailored for those moments when time is of the essence. These time-efficient routines will keep you on track, ensuring that you never have to compromise your commitment to fitness.

Whether you're a busy professional, a dedicated parent, or juggling multiple responsibilities, these tips and quick Pilates workouts are designed to empower you to stay on the path of wellness. Let's break the cycle of starting and stopping, and instead, forge a sustainable and enduring relationship with Pilates that aligns with your bustling lifestyle. Together, let's make consistent progress toward a stronger, healthier, and more confident you!

How to Stay Consistent

Getting started on any kind of fitness journey is a commitment to personal well-being, and the key to unlocking its full potential lies in unwavering consistency. Wall Pilates, as a results driven practice, demands dedicated and strategic planning to achieve the body you want. Consistency serves as the cornerstone of this journey, providing the framework upon which strength, flexibility, and a well-toned body are built. It is through the repeated engagement with Wall Pilates exercises that the body adapts, evolves, and ultimately transforms.

By fostering a regular and committed practice, individuals not only enhance their physical capabilities but also cultivate a resilient mindset that extends beyond the mat. In the realm of Wall Pilates, consistency is not merely a routine; it is a powerful catalyst propelling individuals toward their fitness goals and nurturing enduring well-being.

Consistency Tips

Set Realistic Goals: Establish achievable short-term and long-term goals. Realistic objectives make it easier to stay motivated and track your progress.

Create a Schedule: Block out dedicated time for Wall Pilates in your daily or weekly schedule. You should treat these appointments with the same level of importance as any other commitment. Find a Workout Buddy: Enlist a friend or family member to join you in your Wall Pilates sessions. Having a workout buddy not only makes it more enjoyable but also provides mutual accountability.

Mix Up Your Routine: Keep things interesting by incorporating a variety of exercises. A diverse routine helps prevent boredom and keeps you engaged.

Reward Yourself: Celebrate your achievements, whether big or small. Rewards can be motivational and reinforce the positive habit of consistent Pilates practice.

Track Your Progress: Maintain a workout journal to document your exercises, sets, and repetitions. Tracking progress provides a visual representation of your journey and serves as a powerful motivator.

Stay Flexible: Life can be unpredictable, and schedules may change. Be adaptable and find alternative times to fit in your Wall Pilates when unexpected events occur.

Utilize Technology: Explore Pilates apps or online platforms that offer guided sessions. Having access to virtual classes allows you to practice Wall Pilates at your convenience.

Create a Dedicated Space: Designate a specific area for your Wall Pilates practice. Having a dedicated space helps signal to your brain that it's time for a workout, promoting consistency.

Prioritize Self-Care: Recognize the importance of self-care and how Wall Pilates contributes to your overall well-being. Make it a non-negotiable part of your self-care routine.

By implementing these tips, you can cultivate a consistent Wall Pilates practice that aligns seamlessly with your lifestyle, fostering a healthier and stronger you over time.

However, recognizing that time constraints are a common challenge, especially in today's fast-paced world, I've curated shorter yet effective Wall Pilates workouts. These quick routines cater to busy schedules, ensuring that even the most time-strapped individuals can infuse their day with the revitalizing benefits of Wall Pilates. It's not always about the duration but the commitment to prioritizing your well-being. These concise workouts serve as a testament that, even in the busiest of days, a few minutes of focused Pilates can make a significant impact on your physical and mental vitality.

So, whether you have a hectic schedule or just need a quick energy boost, these efficient Pilates sessions are designed to keep you consistent on your journey to a stronger, more resilient you.

10-Minute Ab Sculpting Core Blast

The 10-Minute Ab Sculpting Core Blast is designed as a quick yet highly effective routine to fortify and define your abdominal muscles. The carefully selected exercises engage the entire core, including the rectus abdominis, obliques, and lower abdominal muscles. The workout begins with a challenging Wall Plank, promoting core stability and endurance. As you transition through Wall Sit Twists, Leg Raises, Oblique Crunches, Wall Mountain Climbers, Reverse Crunches, Bicycle Crunches, and Russian Twists, each movement targets specific areas of your core, enhancing strength and flexibility.

The purpose of this dynamic routine is to intensify core activation, fostering both stability and endurance. Throughout the workout, you should feel a deep engagement in your core muscles, signifying the effectiveness of each exercise. By completing the circuit twice within a 10-minute timeframe, you'll not only experience the burn that comes with optimal activation but also enjoy the sculpting and toning benefits for your entire core. Focus on controlled movements and maintain correct form to maximize the results of this powerful Ab Sculpting Core Blast.

10-Minute Ab Sculpting Core Blast

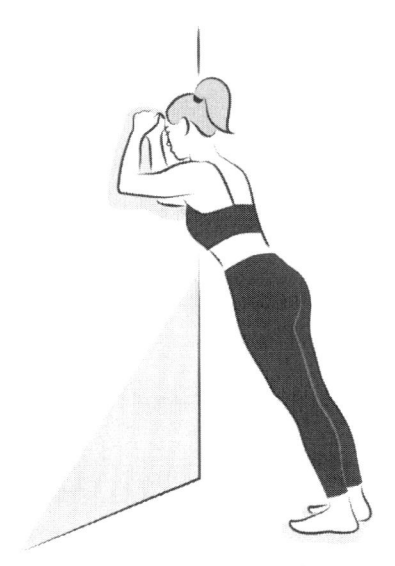

Exercise 1: Wall Plank

Place hands on the wall at shoulder height.

Step back into a plank position, maintaining a straight line from head to heels.

Hold for 30 seconds, engaging your core and keeping a straight line from head to heels.

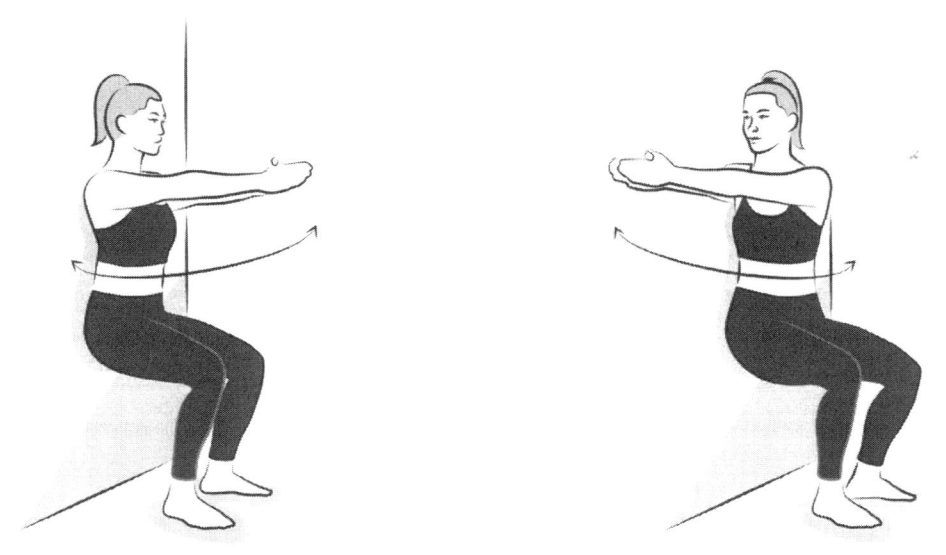

Exercise 2: Wall Sit Twists

Sit against the wall with knees bent at a 90-degree angle.

Place hands together and twist your torso from side to side, reaching towards the wall. Perform 15 twists on each side.

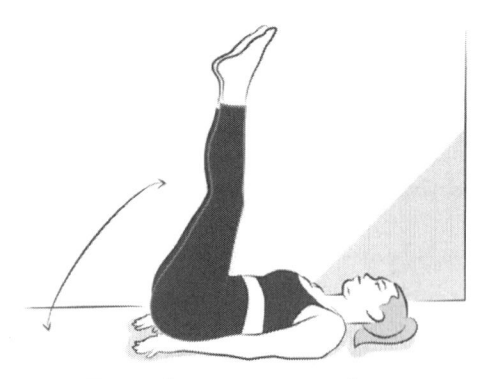

Exercise 3: Leg Raises

Lie on your back, legs against the wall, and hands under your lower back.

Lift your legs towards the ceiling and lower them without touching the floor. Perform 15 reps.

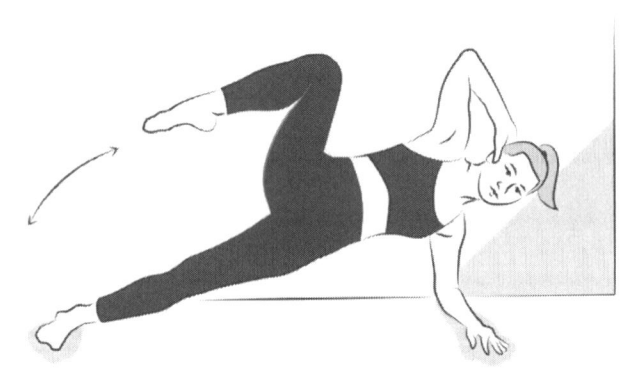

Exercise 4: Oblique Crunches

Lie on your side, with hips and shoulders against the wall.

Place the bottom hand on the floor and the top hand behind your head.

Lift your upper body towards the ceiling, and draw the top leg's knee towards the elbow of the arm that's behind your head to really target the obliques. Perform 12 reps on each side.

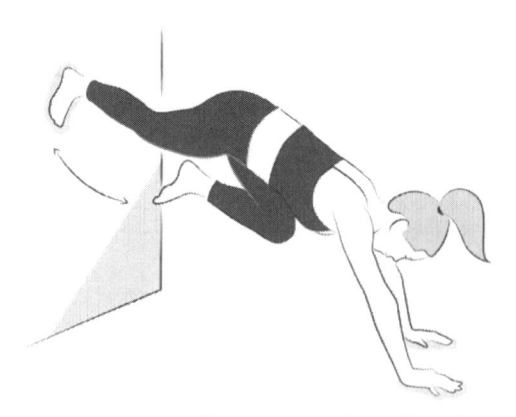

Exercise 5: Wall Mountain Climbers

Get into a plank position with your feet against the wall.

Alternate bringing your knees towards your chest in a running motion. Perform 30 seconds of mountain climbers.

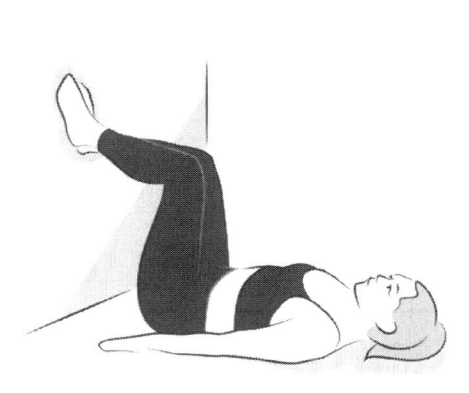

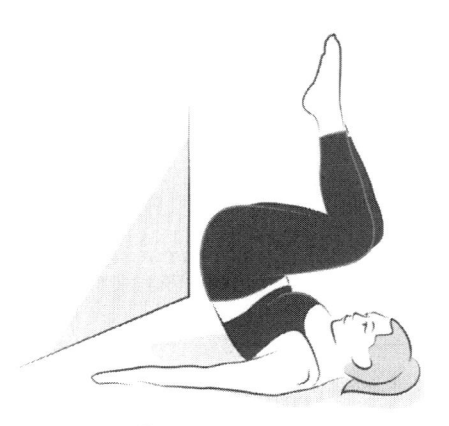

Exercise 6: Reverse Crunches

Lie on your back, hands beside you, and legs raised against the wall.

Lift your hips off the ground towards the ceiling. Perform 15 reps.

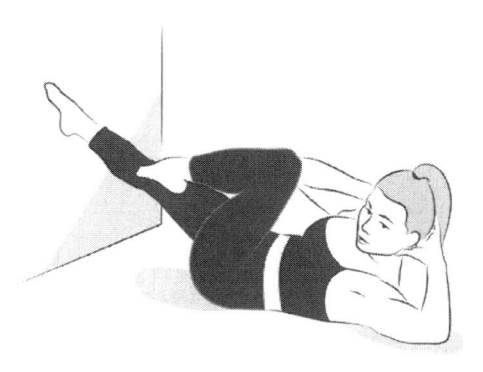

Exercise 7: Bicycle Crunches

Lie on your back, feet against the wall, and hands behind your head.

Bring one knee towards your chest while drawing your abs in. Twist your torso to bring the opposite elbow towards the knee.

Switch sides in a pedaling motion. Perform 20 reps.

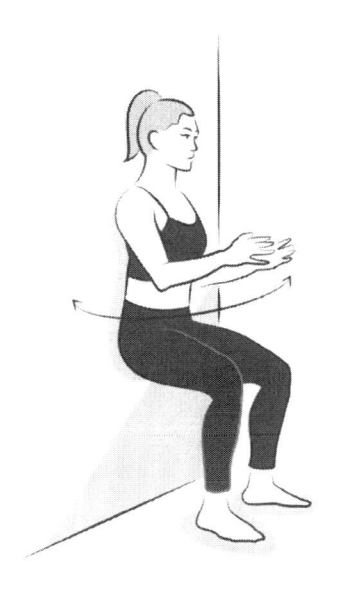

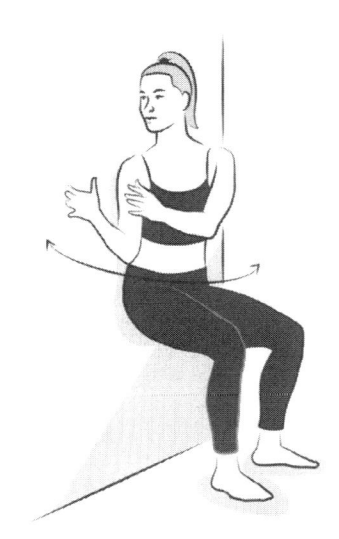

Exercise 8: Russian Twists

Get into a wall-sit position.

Hold your hands, spaced apart in front, with elbows bent and palm facing palm. Now twist the torso from side to side. To Increase difficulty, hold a light weight. Perform 20 twists.

> **Sets and Repetitions**: Complete the circuit twice for a total of 10 minutes.
>
> **Targets**: Engages your entire core, including the rectus abdominis, obliques, and lower abdominal muscles.
>
> **Purpose**: This dynamic core blast aims to enhance core strength, stability, and endurance. It's a quick and effective routine to sculpt and define your abdominal muscles.
>
> **What to Feel**: Expect to feel a deep engagement in your core muscles, promoting a burn that signifies effective activation. Focus on controlled movements and proper form throughout the workout for optimal results.

15-minute Glute-Focused Booty Builder

The 15-Minute Glute Focused Booty Builder is an essential addition to your workout routine, designed to sculpt and lift your glutes for a toned and shapely lower body. Each exercise within this circuit precisely targets the gluteus maximus, medius, and minimus muscles, ensuring a comprehensive engagement for optimal results.

The combination of wall sit booty pulses, wall bridges, wall kicks, wall lunges, wall donkey kicks, wall squats, and wall step-ups creates a dynamic and challenging sequence. By completing this circuit twice in just 15 minutes, you'll experience a targeted burn in your glute muscles, indicating the effective activation and engagement required for a lifted and toned booty.

Focus on controlled movements, maintain correct form, and revel in the sculpting benefits of this purposeful Glute Focused Booty Builder, contributing to both strength and aesthetic appeal in your lower body.

15-minute Glute-Focused Booty Builder

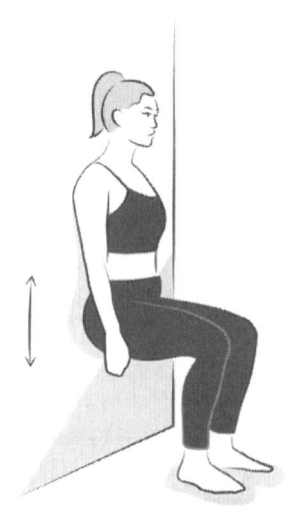

Exercise 1: Wall Sit Booty Pulses

Start with your back against the wall and lower down into a wall sit position.

Pulse your hips up and down, focusing on engaging your glutes. Perform 3 sets of 20 pulses.

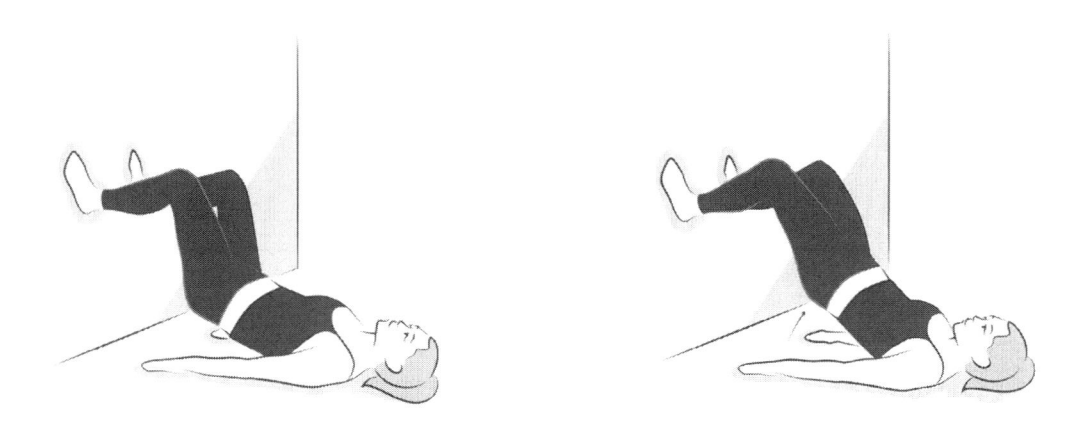

Exercise 2: Wall Bridge

Lie on your back with feet against the wall, knees bent.

Lift hips towards the ceiling, so that your shoulders, hips and knees are in a straight line. Perform 3 sets of 15 repetitions.

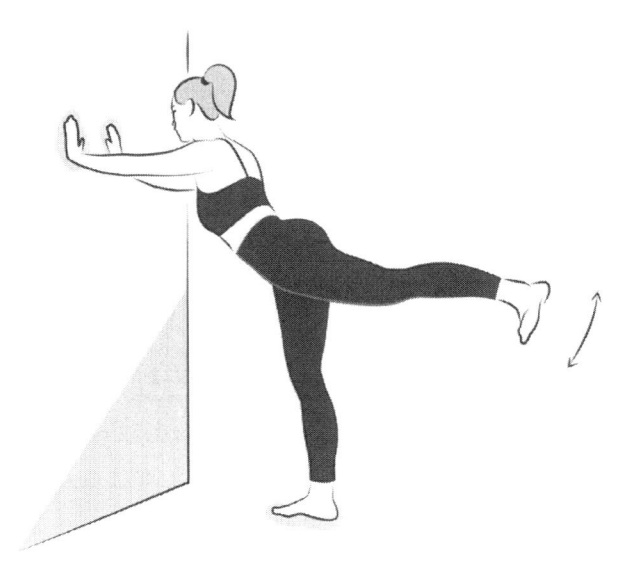

Exercise 3: Wall Kickback

Stand facing the wall, place your hands on the wall for support.

Lift one leg back, keeping it straight, and pulse it towards the ceiling. Perform 2 sets of 20 pulses on each leg.

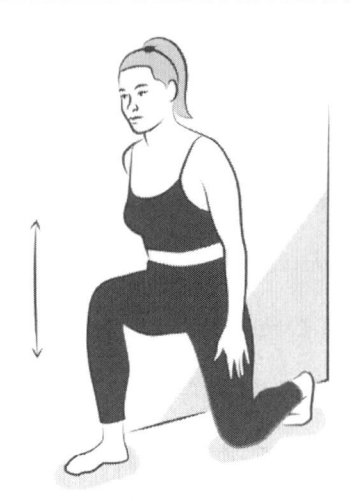

Exercise 4: Lunges

Stand a few feet away from the wall, place one foot against it. Lower into a lunge, keeping your knee directly above your ankle. Push back up to the starting position. Perform 3 sets of 12 lunges on each leg.

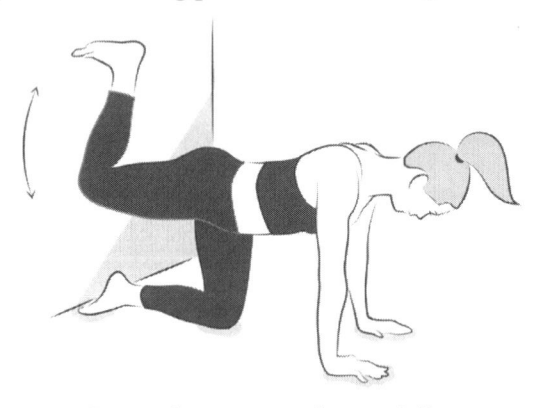

Exercise 5: Donkey Kicks

Start on all fours with your hands on the floor and your toes against the wall. Lift one leg towards the ceiling, focusing on squeezing your glutes. Perform 3 sets of 15 kicks on each leg.

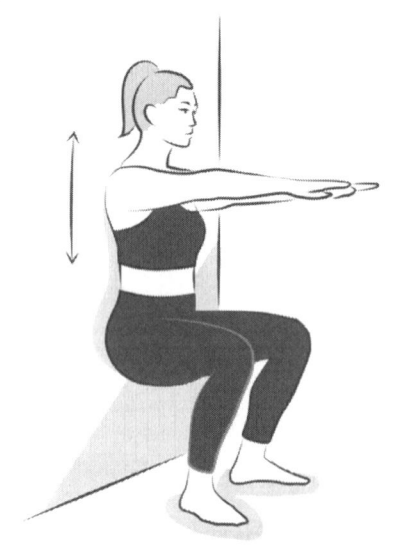

Exercise 6: Wall Squats

Stand with your back against the wall and lower into a squat position. Keep your knees aligned with your ankles. Perform 3 sets of 15 squats.

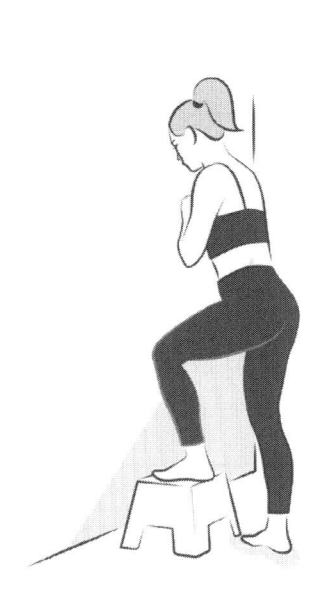

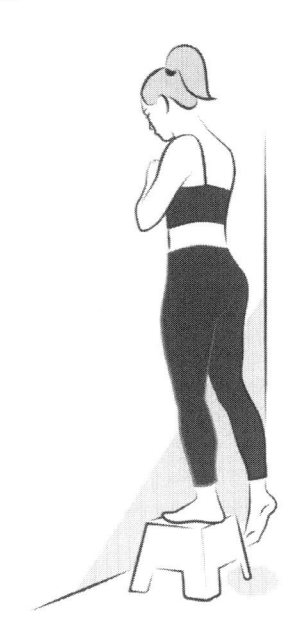

Exercise 7: Step-Ups

Face the wall and step one foot onto a sturdy surface, like a bench or step. Push through your heel to lift your body up, then step back down. Perform 3 sets of 12 step-ups on each leg.

> **Sets and Repetitions**: Complete the circuit twice for a total of 15 minutes.
>
> **Targets**: Engages the glute muscles, including the gluteus maximus, medius, and minimus.
>
> **Purpose**: This Glute-Focused Booty Builder is crafted to tone and lift your glutes, promoting overall lower body strength and aesthetic appeal.
>
> **What to Feel**: Expect to feel a targeted burn in your glute muscles throughout the workout, signifying effective activation and engagement. Focus on controlled movements and maintain proper form to maximize the sculpting and lifting benefits for your booty.

10-Minute Legs and Arms Toning Workout

The 10-Minute Legs and Arms Toning Workout is a versatile routine that efficiently targets both your lower body and arms. The Wall Squats with Bicep Curls engage your quads, hamstrings, and biceps, promoting strength and toning in these muscle groups. Wall Push-Ups work your chest, shoulders, and triceps, enhancing upper body definition and strength. The Wall Lunges with Lateral Raises combine leg toning with an arm workout, ensuring a comprehensive fitness experience. Wall Leg Raises activate your core and lower body.

Completing the circuit twice in just 10 minutes delivers a quick yet effective full-body workout, making it an ideal choice for those with a busy schedule. Expect to feel a satisfying burn in your legs and arms, signifying the targeted engagement that leads to toned and strengthened muscles. Maintain proper form throughout for optimal toning benefits.

10-Minute Legs and Arms Toning Workout

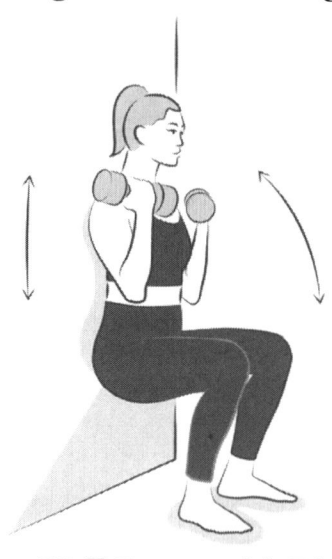

Exercise 1: Wall Squats with Bicep Curls

Stand with your back against the wall and hold dumbbells in each hand, arms at your sides.

Lower into a squat position while simultaneously performing bicep curls.

Push through your heels to return to the starting position. Do 3 sets of 15 reps.

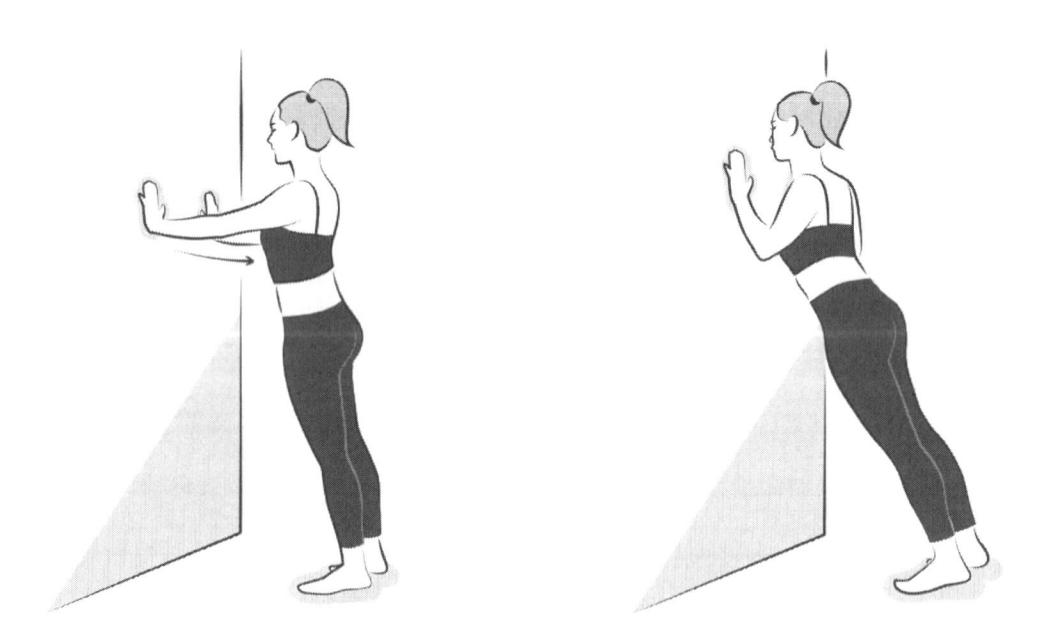

Exercise 2: Wall Push-Ups

Face the wall and place your hands shoulder-width apart.

Perform push-ups by bending your elbows and lowering your chest towards the wall.

Push back up to the starting position. Do 3 sets of 12 reps.

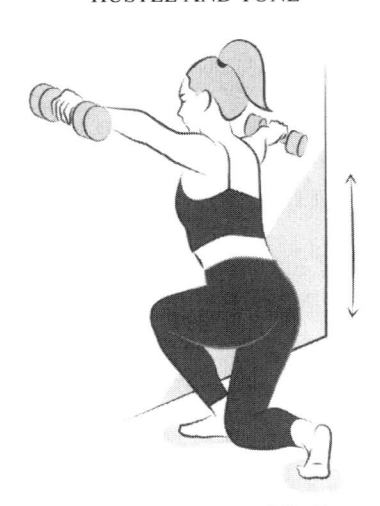

Exercise 3: Cross Lunges with Lateral Raises

Stand facing the wall and hold dumbbells in each hand at your sides.

Step one foot back and across into a lunge while simultaneously raising your arms to the sides. Focus on keeping the hips facing forwards as you move to fully engage the glutes. Push off the back foot to return to the starting position. Do 3 sets of 12 lunges on each leg.

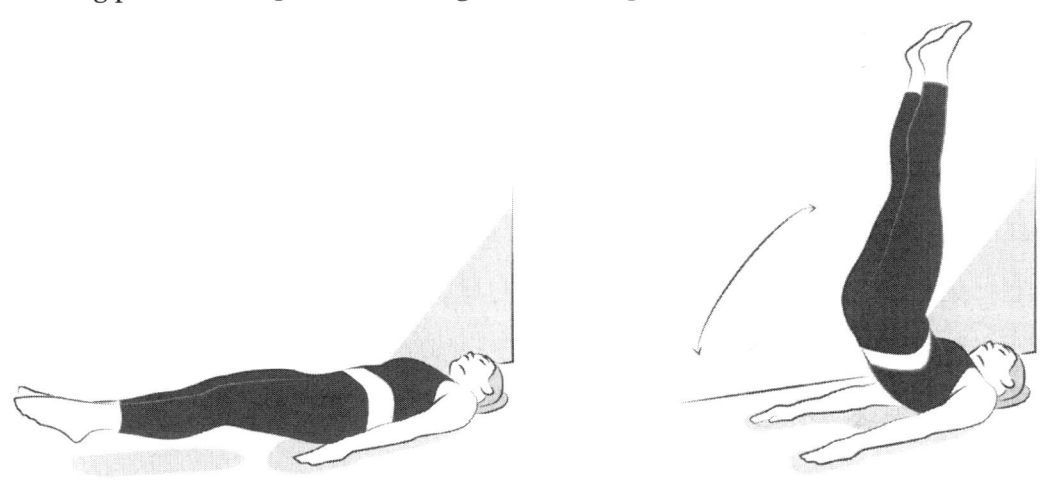

Exercise 4: Leg Raise Crunch

Lie on your back with your legs extended. Lift the legs towards the ceiling. At the top of the motion, lift the hips, pushing the feet upward engaging your core.

Lower the hips to the floor, followed by the legs. Try not to touch the floor with the feet. Do 3 sets of 15 reps.

Sets and Repetitions: Complete the circuit twice for a total of 10 minutes.

Targets: Engages the leg muscles (quads, hamstrings) and arm muscles (biceps, triceps).

Purpose: This Legs and Arms Toning Workout is designed to simultaneously target and tone your lower body and arms, providing a quick and efficient full-body workout.

What to Feel: Anticipate feeling a burn in your legs and arms as you perform each exercise, indicating effective muscle engagement. Maintain proper form throughout the workout to maximize toning benefits.

Other Ways to Use These Quick Workouts

These versatile Wall Pilates workouts, including the 10-Minute Ab Sculpting Core Blast, the 15-Minute Glute Focused Booty Builder, and the 10-Minute Legs and Arms Toning Workout, are not exclusively reserved for those with hectic schedules; they can also serve as valuable extensions to other Pilates routines or complement various forms of exercise. Beyond being quick solutions for individuals on a tight schedule, these workouts can be seamlessly integrated into the end of a Wall Pilates session, providing an effective cool-down and enhancing your core, glutes, and overall body strength.

Moreover, they make excellent companions to activities like long walks, runs, or even yoga sessions, offering a targeted boost to specific muscle groups. Picture incorporating the Ab Sculpting Core Blast after a morning yoga flow or the Legs and Arms Toning Workout following an evening run. The adaptability of these workouts allows you to tailor your fitness routine to different contexts and preferences. Whether you're pressed for time or looking to enhance an existing workout, these Pilates sessions offer a dynamic and efficient way to achieve your fitness goals.

Other Ways to Use These Workouts

Morning Energizer: Kickstart your day with the 10-Minute Ab Sculpting Core Blast to activate your core muscles, promoting focus and vitality.

Lunch Break Booster: Sneak in the 15-Minute Glute Focused Booty Builder during your lunch break to give your glutes a targeted workout, leaving you refreshed for the afternoon.

Post-Work Wall Pilates: Add the 10-Minute Legs and Arms Toning Workout as a finishing touch to your Wall Pilates session, enhancing the overall toning effect.

Afternoon Pick-Me-Up: Combat the midday slump with a quick round of the Ab Sculpting Core Blast to re-energize and engage your abdominal muscles.

Pre-Run Activation: Warm up with the Legs and Arms Toning Workout before a run to activate your leg muscles and improve overall endurance.

Evening Wind Down: Unwind after a long day by incorporating the Glute Focused Booty Builder into your evening routine, promoting relaxation and toning.

Weekend Warrior: Use any of these workouts during the weekend, either individually or combined, for a quick fitness session between errands and social activities.

Yoga Companion: Pair the Ab Sculpting Core Blast with your morning or evening yoga practice for a comprehensive workout targeting core strength.

Post-Walk Toner: After a brisk walk, intensify the impact on your legs and arms with the Legs and Arms Toning Workout.

Quick Circuit: Combine all three workouts for a dynamic circuit, ensuring a full-body workout in a short period, ideal for busy days.

FREE BONUS:

ACCESS YOUR WALL PILATES FULL VIDEO GUIDES HERE!

Amazing work for making it through and learning so many Wall Pilates exercises! I have included full video guides, exercise charts, and the full audiobook for free to help you to always get the most out of your Wall Pilates workouts.

To access these all of these free bonuses, go to your internet browser and type in bit.ly/wall-pilates and I'll email them over to you.

You can also scan the QR Code below with your cell phone camera and tap the little link that appears if you find that easier.

Keep consistent, stay focused, and you'll be amazed at what you can achieve in a relatively short amount of time. And as always, focus on form and listen to your body, and you'll do great.

Before We Conclude Our Journey Together

I have a question to ask you: If it took you less than 60 seconds of your time and cost you nothing, would you be whiling to do me a small favor?

If you would, that's amazing! All you have to do is leave an honest review on Amazon for this book.

Even though the quick and simple act of leaving a review will take you **less than 60 seconds**, it will give a huge amount of support to so many people.

Your review may help someone start the fitness program that they keep putting off. Perhaps it will help empower someone to get in the shape they always wanted, even though they feel too shy to go to a gym. It could help so many people just like you transform themselves from where they are today, to where they want to be.

Your words are powerful, your kindness is amazing, and your time is appreciated.

To make that happen and to keep it quick and simple, scan one of the QR codes with your cell phone's camera and press the link that pops up to go directly to your Amazon review page:

| Review Amazon US | Review Amazon UK | Review Amazon CA |

Or head over to your Amazon app, open the pop up menu (bottom right), click to view your orders, choose the book and select the 'Write a product review' option.

Thank you from the bottom of my heart. I truly appreciate you, I appreciate your time, and you have just made my day.

Your coach, Eva

CONCLUSION

ONE JOURNEY'S END, ANOTHER BEGINNING

"Just believe in yourself. Even if you don't, pretend that you do, and at some point, you will."
- VENUS WILLIAMS

"Can you believe how Pilates has changed our lives?" Lucy, with a smile, says as she applies sunscreen.

The beach breeze tousles our hair as Lucy, Sophia, Heather, and I unfold our colorful beach towels. Laughter fills the air, a symphony of joy echoing our shared Wall Pilates journey.

Sophia chimes in, "Absolutely! I never thought I'd feel this strong and confident."

As we settle in, Heather reflects, "Eva, your guidance made all the difference."

Gratitude fills the space between us.

With a chuckle, I reply, "It's incredible to see how far we've come together!"

Lucy, adjusting her sunglasses, adds with a playful grin, "And can we talk about the bonus of Pilates for bikini season? My abs have never been more toned!"

Sophia nods in agreement, "Seriously, it's like magic for sculpting the perfect beach body."

Heather chimes in, "My friends keep asking what my secret is, and I tell them it's the power of Pilates with Eva!"

As the sun sinks lower on the horizon, casting a golden hue on the sand, we revel in the shared triumphs of our toned bodies and newfound confidence. Pilates has woven a tapestry of strength, laughter, and beauty, transforming our lives and making every beach day a celebration of self-love.

...

Congratulations, dear reader, on reaching the conclusion of this wall Pilates guide! Your commitment and dedication throughout this journey have been truly commendable. As your guide, I want to express how well you've done and acknowledge the significant strides you've made on the path to a healthier, stronger you.

Throughout the chapters, you've learned about the origins and effectiveness of Pilates, learned about the unique aspects of Wall Pilates, and navigated through specifically designed programs. By completing this book, you've not only gained valuable insights into the world of Pilates but have also transformed your body and mindset.

You've set and achieved goals, discovered the benefits of morning and evening routines, and embraced the efficiency of 15-minute wall Pilates sessions. Progressing from the beginner to advanced programs, you've sculpted your body, built confidence, and enhanced your strength. The finishing program marked a culmination of your efforts, possibly introducing weights for an added challenge.

This comprehensive guide has been meticulously crafted to address the specific pain points you've experienced on your fitness journey. Let's look at how this book serves as the solution to each of these challenges.

Achieving a Sculpted Physique

The Intermediate and Advanced Programs introduced in this book strategically target different muscle groups, contributing to the sculpting of your arms, legs, and, yes, that coveted bigger butt. The carefully curated exercises aim to create a goddess-like physique, enhancing your overall aesthetic appeal.

Weight Loss and Fat Burning

The wall Pilates routines provided here focus on dynamic movements that engage various muscle groups, effectively aiding weight loss and reducing body fat. Specifically designed exercises target common problem areas such as the stomach, arms, and back, helping you shed unwanted pounds while toning your physique.

Enhancing Strength, Flexibility, and Body Confidence

Through a progressive approach in the Beginner, Intermediate, and Advanced Programs, this book systematically builds strength and flexibility. The incorporation of wall Pilates exercises fosters a balanced, firm body while preserving a feminine aesthetic. As you witness your physical capabilities expand, your body confidence will naturally soar.

As you stand at the conclusion of this our journey together, I want to encourage you to keep forging ahead. Your achievements thus far are a testament to your strength and commitment. Take a moment to reflect on how far you've come, and let that sense of accomplishment fuel your determination for the journey ahead.

Set new and more demanding goals, and challenge yourself with higher intensity, so you can hit your next 28-day program with confidence. You've already demonstrated incredible commitment, and I have no doubt that you'll continue to push yourself to achieve more than you ever thought possible.

All types of self-improvement at first takes a goal, then undeterred dedication, and finally it takes action to truly unlock the results that you desire. By following the programs in this book from start to finish, your efforts have been truly inspiring.

CONCLUSION

Key Takeaways

Goal Setting: Understand the importance of setting personal goals for your Wall Pilates journey. Goals provide direction, motivation, and a sense of accomplishment.

Mind-Body Connection: Emphasize the significance of connecting with your breath and maintaining mindfulness during workouts. This connection enhances your overall Pilates experience.

Warm-Up and Cool-Down: Recognize the value of proper warm-up and cool-down routines. These practices contribute to improved workout performance, faster recovery, and enhanced muscle quality.

Structured Programs: Follow the meticulously designed Beginner, Intermediate, and Advanced Programs, each progressing in intensity. Consistency is key to seeing lasting results.

Variety in Routines: Explore different routines, including morning and evening sessions, as well as quick 15-minute workouts. This variety accommodates various schedules and keeps your Pilates journey dynamic.

Gradual Progression: As you advance, embrace progressions that challenge you further, even moving away from the wall. Listen to your body and prioritize safety to avoid injury.

Celebrating Achievements: Congratulate yourself on the achievements gained throughout the book. Acknowledge your increased strength, sculpted physique, boosted confidence, and overall wellness.

Now, armed with the knowledge and practical experience gained from this book, it's time to take action. Apply the principles, techniques, and routines you've learned in your daily life. Set new goals, challenge yourself, and continue the journey toward a healthier, more empowered you.

Before we conclude, I'd like to remind you on more time that consistency is the key to lasting success. Whether you're a Wall Pilates enthusiast or a just getting started on your fitness journey, each day is an opportunity to progress further. Take charge of your goals, and use the power of Wall Pilates to achieve the results that you want and earn the body that you deserve.

There was never any doubt in my mind about how well you would do, and here you are, a testament to your unwavering commitment. Your journey doesn't end here; it evolves into new challenges and triumphs.

As you venture forward, I want you to know I'm cheering you on every step of the way. The book may end, but your journey towards strength, vitality, and a well sculpted physique continues.

Here's to your ongoing success, and well-being!

References

"6 Ways to Increase Intensity of Your Pilates Exercise!" Pilates Plus, 20 Sept. 2021, pilatesplus.sg/6-ways-to-increase-intensity-of-your-pilates-exercise/#:~:text=The%20Intensity%20of%20a%20Pilates,working%20on%20a%20proper%20technique.

"7 Minutes of This Bedtime Wall Pilates Will Make You Sleep Like A Baby!" YouTube, YouTube, 29 June 2023, https://www.youtube.com/watch?v=yXU9dA01PuQ. Accessed 19 Jan. 2024.

"28 Day Wall Pilates Challenge for Beginners | Build Core Strength at Home!" YouTube, YouTube, 4 June 2023, https://www.youtube.com/watch?v=CpO-oY4fpiQ. Accessed 19 Jan. 2024.

Balcetis, Emily. " Why Some People Find Exercise Harder than Others." Jesmond Pool & Gym, TedTalks, 25 Feb. 2021, jesmondpool.online/9-motivating-and-inspiring-ted-talks-on-fitness-exercise-and-wellbeing/.

Benshosan, April. "Best Pilates Warm-up Exercises ." LIVESTRONG.COM, Leaf Group, www.livestrong.com/article/452300-pilates-warm-up-exercises/. Accessed 19 Jan. 2024.

Carolan, Julie. "Benefits of Morning Pilates." Julie Carolan Physical Therapy & Pilates, 19 Feb. 2019, www.treaturcore.com/benefits-of-morning-pilates/.

Collins, Jenna, director. 15 Min Full Body WALL PILATES | Burn Fat & Tone Up. YouTube, YouTube, 8 Nov. 2023, https://www.youtube.com/watch?v=N9h7F04aAuM. Accessed 19 Jan. 2024.

Page, Danielle. "People Are Raving about Wall Pilates for Fast Results. Does It Really Work?" TODAY.Com, Today Show, www.today.com/health/diet-fitness/wall-pilates-exercises-rcna103846. Accessed 3 Feb. 2024.

Marguerite Ogle MS, RYT. "Advanced Pilates Exercises on the Mat." Verywell Fit, Verywell Fit, 24 June 2019, www.verywellfit.com/advanced-pilates-exercises-on-the-mat-2704716.

McKee, Liz. "10 Top Tips for Your Morning Pilates Routine." LSF Pilates Studio, LSF Pilates Studio, 27 Dec. 2020, www.lsfpilates.com/blog/2020/12/27/10-top-tips-for-your-morning-pilates-routine.

Mukhwana, Jeremy. "Wall Pilates Program to Activate Your Body's Natural Movement Patterns." BetterMe Blog, 26 Oct. 2023, betterme.world/articles/wall-pilates-program/.

Mukhwana, Jeremy. "The Pros and Cons of Pilates vs. Weight Training." BetterMe Blog, 1 May 2023, betterme.world/articles/pilates-vs-weight-training/.

Porter, Alice. "This 15-Minutes Wall Pilates Routine Will Help You Build Strength While Protecting Your Joints." Yahoo!, Fit & Well, www.yahoo.com/lifestyle/15-minutes-wall-pilates-routine-060039615.html. Accessed 27 Jan. 2024.

Phitosophy. "6 Best Warm up Exercises before Pilates Class." Phit, 11 Oct. 2023, www.phitosophy.com/6-best-warm-up-exercises-before-pilates-class/.

"Pilates and Breathwork: Understanding the Importance of Breath in Your." Pilates Reformers Plus, pilatesreformersplus.com/blogs/news/pilates-and-breathwork-understanding-the-importance-of-breath-in-your-practice#:~:text=By%20consciously%20linking%20your%20breath,physical%20movements%20and%20mental%20focus. Accessed 19 Jan. 2024.

Sutton, Joanne. "How Do You Fit Pilates into Your Tight Schedule?" *LinkedIn*, 31 Jan. 2022, www.linkedin.com/pulse/how-do-you-fit-pilates-your-tight-schedule-joanne-sutton-/?trk=articles_directory.

Wharton, Chris, director. The Exercise Happiness Paradox . YouTube, YouTube, 30 Sept. 2021, https://www.youtube.com/watch?v=8s01WZ4j10Q. Accessed 19 Jan. 2024.

Printed in Great Britain
by Amazon